Jimmy Golden. MY GOLDEN N
EPILEPSY AND BRAIN SURGEF

Chapter 1. The beginning.

Writing a book about my experience with epilepsy and brain surgery feels kind of strange, and if I can be honest, very unlikely. If someone would have asked me, maybe five years ago, "Hey Jimmy, what do you think is more likely, for you to have brain surgery, or for you to write a book?" I would have most certainly laughed, then came up with some sort of sarcastic answer that allowed me to say neither. I am no author, or at least I wasn't until now. I am an aerospace technician, and an ex law enforcement officer. Before epilepsy entered my life, I was perfectly healthy. I had no reason to believe anything like this would ever happen to me. As soon someone gets to know epilepsy though, they start to realize that it is somewhat different for everyone. Also, it doesn't always have an identifiable cause. It sometimes chooses people like random winners of a dark, unlucky lottery. One in which the player didn't sign up for, for reasons no one, including the doctors battling the disorder can always fully explain. In fact, that seems to be a very hard hitting and powerful lesson. At least that is what I have come to accept while on my journey through epilepsy. It doesn't quite matter if you are the one inflicted with the disorder, if you are a loved one, a friend, a doctor, a med student, or just someone loosely involved with someone who has epilepsy. You will realize that it manifests differently in different people. There may be similarities between us, but no two of our cases seem to be identical. Our stories are all a little different. Our seizures vary in types, in severity, in lengths, and in manifestations. Some of our seizures give warning signs, or auras, while others do not. Some of us have family, friends and or colleagues who are dedicated and devoted to helping and supporting us through our difficult journeys, some of us do not. Some of us have triggers that cause our seizures to begin, almost as if having a start switch, and for others, they just happen, out of nowhere. They are like a silent predator, always watching, always stalking, and we never know when, where, or how vicious the attack is going to be, so we are forced to live our life in a state of perpetual concern and readiness. A state of hyper alert. Some of us and our love ones are ready, willing and eager to work with doctors, and are willing to go through with aggressive and potentially life changing, yet sometimes frightening treatment options like brain surgery. Some are not. I hope that by writing this book, I can give people the courage they need to take interest in those life changing options.

If I asked you to guess, as the reader, about my first experience with seizures, I would be willing to bet it was not what you would imagine for someone like me with epilepsy. I remember the first time the disorder of epilepsy touched my life. I was at work. I was completing some state mandated paperwork when I heard what is considered a cry for help in the setting in which I worked. "Man down! Man down! Man down!" I jumped up, raced out of my office and listened intently to try and see where the desperate cry for help was coming from. The building erupted with noise. It became incredibly loud, which was not necessarily abnormal for the building I was working in, but this was a different kind of loud. It was a frantic and more coordinated kind of noise than was usual for that type of setting. Once I was out of my office, I listened through the noise. The yelling and banging of hands on steel doors is surprisingly loud in those housing units. I could make out someone screaming a door number to me. I ran over to the door. I can still, to this day, hear the sound in my mind of my keys banging around on my duty belt as I ran across the day-room floor. "Clash, clash, clash, clash, clash". In that moment, when I got to the glass of the cell door of the state penitentiary I worked in as a correctional officer, is when I first experienced the darkness of epilepsy. "C.O Golden! My Cell mate is having a seizure!!" I looked through the dirty glass of the cell door, and saw the inmate, lying on the ground, foaming at the mouth, eyes rolled back in his head, violently convulsing. I instructed his cell mate to roll him on his side, put a pillow under his head and to not put anything in his mouth. I activated the building's emergency alarm system. (due to the security level of the building, I was legally unable to open the door until more staff arrived). I got on my radio. "Central control, Alpha 5 floor, be advised, I have a code 1 medical in Alfa 5, cell 1XX, I need Mary 3 at this location, Alpha 5 floor clear". It is difficult to communicate, both through the radio, and in person, with the wailing sound of a state prison's building alarm sounding in the dead of night, but I got my response from central control over the radio. "Attention on institutional grounds, we have a personal alarm activation in Alpha 5, all non-responding units maintain radio silence". Help was on its way. Within seconds of the confirmation of my alarm activation, the tonic-clonic phase of his seizure had passed, and his cell mate stood up and spoke to me. "He has epilepsy". I had heard of it, they prepared us for seizures in the academy, which is why I had instructed his cell mate to do what I did, but I had never witnessed it before. Even as a law enforcement officer, working in a maximum-security prison, who had witnessed some violent, bizarre and even sad things, seeing someone have a tonic-clonic seizure for the first time was certainly a memorable experience. It is brutal. It is not pleasant to watch. Within 30 seconds or less, my backup had arrived on scene, and the ambulance was there shortly after. We got him carefully loaded up and sent him to be taken care of. This was one of many experiences like this I dealt with while doing this job, all while never guessing, one day, soon, I would be the one being loaded into an ambulance after a tonic-clonic seizure, my fiancée, being the one taking care of me and calling for an ambulance. Oh, how things have changed.

I remember my own first seizure quite well. I should say, I remember the beginning and aftermath of it. I was at work, where I work in the aerospace industry now. After being given several advanced potential layoff warning notices, shortly after joining the Department of Corrections, I hesitantly turned in my badge, and resigned from my short-lived career in law enforcement. I went back into aerospace. They had offered me my old job back, and I simply could not refuse with the potential layoff hanging over my head at the time. On the day of my first seizure, I had just gone to lunch. I had, for quite some time been thinking of going back to the California Department of Corrections because the state's financial crisis had cleared up. The fact that I had already been an officer, made the process very easy, and I had been fast tracked up until that point, and the future of the process looked good as well. I was torn about it, because I love my job where I am. I remember that being heavy on my mind that day. I had sat down to eat lunch, and was doing some math in my head about how much PTO, or paid time off, I would have left if I used a day to go through the next step of the hiring process for going back to corrections. Suddenly, I had this extraordinary strange feeling that I had never experienced before, while attempting to do that math in my mind. I still remember the visual mental picture of looking at my lunch box while it happened. Then I remember this tremendous feeling of déjà vu, the likes of which I had never experienced in all my life. It was weird, it was dreamlike. I really felt as if I "knew" that what I was experiencing had already happened, and I was re-living it somehow. It was so strange, I couldn't understand it. Then suddenly, a rush. I had a feeling I can't accurately explain. A type of uprising sensation. Almost the sensation of water flowing on your skin, or wind softly blowing over your body, mixed with soft electricity, mixed with a light burning sensation. It was the strangest feeling I had ever experienced. It was uncomfortable, yet, in a way, it was almost enjoyable, strangely enough. It was as if my emotion center didn't know what to think. After it passed, I thought to myself that I must have been daydreaming or something, because I had been there longer than seemed possible, and I felt strangely out of it and confused. I also felt sick. In fact, I felt so sick I nearly went home. Looking back now, I realize I had lost cognition and had lost time sitting there during that first complex partial seizure that day, and that is why I felt that I must have been day dreaming. I ended up staying at work, wondering why I felt so ill, and wondering what had happened to me. Being who I am though, I passed it off, and thought little of it. I went about my business. Little did I know; my whole life had just changed.

My second seizure happened soon after. About a week after my first seizure, again, while at work. I was on a computer, when again, I started to feel those complex strange feelings. I had been thinking about them since the first one happened, so when the first sign of it arose, I was hyper sensitive of it and was paying attention. I noticed that my left hand and forearm seemed to feel a little twitchy after the original déjà vu had passed. It was as if they attempted to move a little, like my hand was trying to "grasp", open and closed, and I had noticed more of the burning feeling in it. I won't pretend I still wasn't concerned. It was weird. It was uncomfortable. I wasn't sure what to do. I thought about it. At this point though, I didn't really tell anyone. I was afraid to worry people. I thought to myself "if this continues, I will do something about it." At the same time, I was thinking that burning in the left arm and feeling sick after, can be questionable. I really wouldn't even know how to explain the other things though. I had some thinking to do.

Before I knew it, these things were starting to happen more and more. I was starting to become really concerned. I was starting to think that it was time to do something. Maybe something really was wrong or happening to me. I was going to have to talk to someone about it. It was time. The "episodes", as I had taken up to calling them, had seemed to be progressing a little. What I mean by that, is they seemed to have become more intense, or stronger in a way. The feelings they were producing were stronger, the effects they were having on my body were more intense. So, I decided to tell my fiancée.

Jimmy Golden. MY GOLDEN MIND, A JOURNEY THROUGH EPILEPSY AND BRAIN SURGERY

I still remember talking to her. I really didn't know what to say, or even how to say it honestly. After all, I didn't know how to describe it. I really didn't even know what I was setting out to accomplish. I didn't even know what I thought about it at that point. Did I even want to see a doctor? Did I think it was necessary? I was a little concerned, yeah, but at the same time, I was also concerned that going to the doctor and bringing something up, that may be nothing, may disqualify me from going back into law enforcement. Looking back now, that seems like nonsense. Hindsight is 20/20 as they say, but your health is always most important. I had really decided I needed to talk to my fiancée Christina, who, by the way, was not yet my fiancée at the time, because I felt like not telling her was dishonest at that point. There was obviously something going on with me. I had decided that if something like that had been going on with her, that I would hope that she would come to me with it, so we could work through it together. That is what really made me decide to talk to her. So, one day in the kitchen, I was leaning against the sink, and I brought it up to her. I basically said "Christina, I need to bring something up, it's nothing bad about us or anything of course, but there has been something going on with me. It is really difficult to explain, but I have been having these "episodes" for lack of better words, that I can't really explain." I went on to do my best to explain what I had been feeling and experiencing. She, of course, as any concerned loved one would advise, told me I needed to see a doctor. I told her I was worried about how it might cause problems with my career with the Department of Corrections, and of course, she told me how my health is more important. We decided together that it was time.

Jimmy Golden. MY GOLDEN MIND, A JOURNEY THROUGH EPILEPSY AND BRAIN SURGERY

Chapter 2. Time for help.

I had assumed that whatever was going on was likely brain related, pretty much from the start, but, of course, I was not sure. I am science minded and inquisitive by nature, so whenever something comes up that I am curious about, I tend to research it. It didn't take me too long to stumble across the idea that I may be experiencing something that I had never heard of before. Complex partial seizures. The way I had come across this was simple enough. I had googled 'strong, random, strange episodes of déjà vu, weird sensations and loss of cognition.' Before long, I came up with these types of seizures. I was interested, and honestly, a little nervous. I remember thinking, "could I seriously be having seizures?" "No way." "Why would I be?" I couldn't think of any good reason. That was for the doctors to figure out, that was for sure. I was just looking to get a heads up I guess. Maybe even to brace myself in case it was something traumatic. I wondered what kind of process they would put me through. What was going to happen when I told them about all the bizarre things I had been experiencing. It was a little intimidating telling a healthcare professional, at least for me, that I had been having some of these strange feelings, that seemed to be tied to emotions. I guess, maybe, in a way, I worried they would wonder if it was a psychological disorder of some kind. Maybe, deep down, I worried it could be myself. They were, after all, very, very strange. I had no Idea that they were just getting started.

    I remember walking out of the doctor's office after getting my referral to the neurologist, thinking to myself "wow, that was much easier than I thought it would be, I probably should have done this a lot sooner." They didn't give me a hard time at all. They basically just told me that it sounded to them like a neurological issue and that they were going to send me to the neurologist. Awesome! I felt like I was "headed" in the right direction, pun intended.

It didn't take long. I got a call to schedule an appointment with a neurologist. It couldn't come any sooner as far as I was concerned. The episodes were happening more and more frequently at that point. They were not letting up at all. They were strange. The one good thing that seemed to come with time, is that the more episodes I had, the less sick I seemed to feel after having them. I would feel tired and often confused or disoriented to a point depending on the severity, but the more I had, the less sick I felt. As far as the confusion and disorientation went, it was difficult for me to tell just how confused or disoriented I really was. During all this time, because of the nature of my episodes, most people didn't really notice them because I would go into an "autopilot" kind of mode during them. I would basically continue doing whatever I was doing prior to it starting, as if I were not having one. The only exceptions were if I were speaking or having social interactions of any kind. For example, if I was working on something, I would continue to work, If I was walking, I would continue to walk, If I was cleaning, I would continue to clean. It seemed, at first, the only time people would notice something was off, is if I had one when they were having a direct conversation with me, and most of the time, they brushed it off as if I were daydreaming, or just simply as if I had gotten distracted.

I went and saw the neurologist. I was happy that it was finally time. I remember waiting with Christina in the waiting area, and wondering to myself what he would say. The visit was interesting. He did what seemed to be some basic neurological testing after asking me about what was going on. He told me he was going to order an MRI for me. He also said I did fine on the tests that he performed in the office setting. He didn't mention seizures or epilepsy during the visit. Looking back, and after learning everything I have learned throughout my journey through epilepsy, I would like to offer my first piece of advice of this book. Do not be afraid to speak up or mention things to your doctor. If you think that you might have an idea that your doctor may be missing, don't be afraid to bring it up to them. A good doctor will create a bond with you or your loved one and will work with you or them as a team. They will, of course, lead that team, and be the one to guide you to success, and, naturally have most of the knowledge and know how to help you on your road to improving your quality of life when compared to what you, as a random untrained person, would typically have to offer. Sometimes though, what you offer, just might bring something to the table. It could spark an idea. It could help. Bring it up if you find it to be reasonable in your mind and you are curious about it. It couldn't hurt. A doctor should listen about what you believe may be wrong. If they believe you're wrong, they should give you a scientific or rational explanation for their stance. This is especially important when they do not have an answer for what is happening with you. If not, they are waving a red flag. Part of being a good health care provider is providing the patient with education about what is happening to, or within their body.

Although, after reading what I just wrote, you may be able to guess that I shouldn't have, I left my first neurology appointment satisfied enough. Christina, on the other hand, seemed skeptical. She just had an "off" feeling. I will give her credit there. Anyway, I waited for my MRI, which came up rather quickly per the request of the neurologist. I remember, the feeling of having to have my brain scanned was slightly scary. The neurologist had basically said he was doing it to make sure that there was "nothing in there." Let your imagination run wild with that while waiting for an MRI to be taken of your brain, and then while waiting for the results, and you can imagine how uncomfortable that can be, especially with how weird things have been. All kinds of things start running through your mind. I mean, if the neurologist wants to see if there is something in there, does that mean that what I am experiencing are symptoms of something being in there?

I got slightly concerned after getting to work, and had time to think about it. He had ordered the MRI to be done as soon as possible at the imaging center in town. I got a phone call, which I had missed because my phone was outside in my lunch box, and I listened to the voice mail and called them back as soon as I got out there. They wanted me to come in that day, and be there by 4:00pm. If I were to make that appointment, I was going to have to leave work a few minutes early to be safe, but I told them no problem, I was having an MRI done of my brain after all. I was sure my boss would understand. I didn't want to lose the open appointment slot they happened to have. So, I accepted it.

I still remember the conversation. "Hey boss, can I speak with you for a minute?" He replied, "Yeah, what can I do for you Jim?" I said, "Hey man, I have been having some problems, I'm really not sure what is going on yet, but I have to have a brain MRI done, and they just called and want to do it right away. For me to get there, I am going to have to leave about 10 minutes early. I'm sorry, is that cool?". I honestly fully expected him to be worried about me, especially considering it was involving my brain, but he caught me off guard. He sneered at me and said "yeah, fine, go, but next time, you had better give me more notice than this!" Then he stormed off. I thought he was joking and was going to come back and tell me he hoped everything was okay, but he didn't, he was serious. He didn't care. That was the first time I experienced someone being cold hearted about my disorder, although it didn't directly have to do with epilepsy of course. I shouldn't have been surprised though. He honestly was not a very nice person, sad to say. You never know, maybe he was battling his own battles. He ended up being terminated after a while. I doubt I will ever see the man again.

After the day arrived and passed for me to receive MRI results, I didn't hear anything. I waited a little bit. I had wanted to talk to the neurologist anyway, because my episodes had become worse. I was starting to have visual distortions, and or what seemed like hallucinations during them. It was really starting to frighten me. I remember one of them very vividly. I started feeling all the usual feelings and emotions, so I knew that the episode was coming. During the following sensations phase, in front of my face, what seemed to be about three or maybe four arm lengths in front of me, I saw what appeared to be a large pinwheel of different colors. It appeared to be floating in the air and rotating. It seemed solid, as if I could reach up and touch it, and to me, looked as real as anything else I could see. I remember looking at it in amazement wondering how and why it was there. I just stared and watched it spin, until eventually, it dissipated. I noticed myself gripping my left-hand open and closed over and over, which is something that I had noticed more and more often at the end of my episodes, among other things.

Jimmy Golden. MY GOLDEN MIND, A JOURNEY THROUGH EPILEPSY AND BRAIN SURGERY

During another one of my episodes, I was at a stereo shop with a friend, talking to a salesman. I had started to feel the feelings build up inside of me. It was coming. I began to not be able to speak. I lost my words. The way I have found to best describe this inability to speak, is once my brains language center ceases to function, when I attempt to speak, it's not that I physically can't, it's as if my brain no longer knows how to go about the task of language at all. The same as if I were to look at someone and ask them to move something by using only their brain. They simply could not do it, and they would not even know how to begin to attempt to do it. That is how it feels when sections become overrun by the electrical storm of brain activity during a seizure. It's not that you can't do the tasks physically, it's that you no longer have the mental capacity to even know where to begin, as if that section of brain that controls those functions no longer exists.

After my language shut down on this poor, unsuspecting, and probably at that point, uncomfortable salesman, I remember staring at him and feeling the feelings of déjà vu. What happened next, was up to that point, the most frightening thing I had experienced with my undiagnosed epilepsy. The man, who I was blankly staring at, presumably unresponsively, started, for lack of better explanation, from my perspective, melting. The distortions started on what would be his left cheek. It is ingrained in my memory. His face started drooping and stretching like heated wax. First, just on that side, then his entire face, like something in a horror movie. His mouth stretched down and open, and his eyes drooped down and sagged. I very vaguely remember stepping back at that point and plopping down into the chairs along the wall behind me. The next thing I remember is wandering around outside, regaining cognition and seeing my friend, who had been waiting in the truck. This friend of mine, Aldo, is one of the few people that I had told about my "episodes". He is one of my dearest friends in life. I told him when I regained cognition, that I had just had another one of "those episodes" that I was recently telling him about. He had just missed my lack of cognition, although I am sure he could see my slight state of disorientation. He asked if I was okay, and after telling him I was, I thought about the salesman inside. I thought he probably thought I was rude, or, who knows what.

Jimmy Golden. MY GOLDEN MIND, A JOURNEY THROUGH EPILEPSY AND BRAIN SURGERY

So, I decided I had better go back in and try and explain to him what was going on. He was very understanding. I apologized to him. I told him that I had been having some strange episodes recently, and I am not quite sure what exactly just happened because I don't remember everything, but I remember enough to know that I just had one, and it was weird, and I know I was probably acting strange, and whatever I did, I meant no disrespect. I told him I was seeing a neurologist about it, and had hope that he would get it figured out for me, because I wasn't much of a fan of what was going on. He told me not to worry about it, he could tell that I seemed off, and he figured I was not feeling well. He didn't take it personally. I appreciated it. He treated me much better than my boss after all. After that, I decided to go with them for all my stereo needs from then on out. I still do to this day.

When Aldo and I left the store that day, I talked to him about it. As I have already said, him and I had discussed the problem before, but that was the most disturbing episode I had ever had, so I was glad he was there with me to talk about it. Before I explained the episode, I told him I didn't know what to think anymore. I told him I felt like I could honestly be losing my mind. I told him, frankly, I was a little bit afraid. Then I explained what it was like. We both seemed to agree that it was time for me to get back in contact with the neurologist and tell him that they were getting worse. Up until that point, I had still been waiting for him to call with the results from my MRI, which still had never come.

"She told you what!" Christina was blown away. I couldn't believe it either. I had contacted my neurologist's office to request a new appointment. When they called me back, his nurse informed me that the Neurologist had received my MRI results, and they were clear. I had no abnormalities. Everything was good, so he didn't need to see me. I told her that was great news, but I still really needed to talk to him because things were getting worse, something was wrong, so I needed to update him and see what to do and where to go from there. She told me she would talk to him and call me back. Not too long later, she called me back and she told me "Dr. ---------- wanted me to inform you, again, that he reviewed your MRI results, and there are no abnormalities, so he DOES NOT need to see you at this time." I told her that I understood that the MRI was clean, but I needed to see him because there was still something wrong with me, and things have changed, my symptoms have changed, I have new things to report. She flat out told me no. I couldn't believe it. I was at a loss for words, I didn't know what to do, she hung up.

Later, Christina and I decided what was best would be to schedule an appointment with my primary care physician. We really didn't know what else to do. He had a relatively soon appointment available, so I got in as soon as I could, suffering through as few episodes along the way as possible. When I saw him that day, I told him what had been going on, the best I could that is. It's funny really. I find myself snickering a little when I think about that line. If you have epilepsy, and you are reading this book, you will understand why. It really is almost impossible, isn't it? To explain them? If you ever find a good way to explain the way they feel, publish it! Anyway, as I was saying, I did my best to explain what was happening to me, and the first thing he said was "well, if you hadn't already had a MRI done, the first thing I would honestly think is that you could possibly have a tumor, but since that is clean, you really need to continue seeing your neurologist. This definitely seems to be a neurological issue, at least to me." I told him what had happened, and that the neurologist had refused to see me. His eyebrows raised in astonishment. He told me he couldn't believe that he had done that to me. He said that it seemed wrong to him for a doctor to do that to someone. "I will tell you what I will do Jimmy, I will write you a new referral to see him again. That way he will HAVE to see you." That was awesome. My first taste of having a doctor who cared about my well-being through this long journey I have been on. In fact, now that this is fresh in my mind because of this book, the next time I see him, I am going to shake his hand and thank him for doing that for me. He is a good man.

My next visit with my neurologist seemed to be more of the same. He seemed to kind of put me through the same standard tests again, like he had every time I had visited him. It was more like visiting a chiropractor than a neurologist, if that makes sense. Not that I have any issue with chiropractors, I mean that in the sense of sort of going through a bit of an actual physical routine, as appose to doing the diagnostic type of work you would expect when someone is in the situation I was in. More red flags I seemed to be ignoring, for reasons I still can't quite fathom to this day. That time though, I told him of the changes. I told him how extreme the episodes were getting. I explained some of them to him. That time, I even brought up the complex partial seizure topic I had read about online. He told me he did not believe I was having seizures. I pressed the issue a little bit because I felt as though he was brushing it off and was not explaining anything to me. He told me if it would make me feel better, he would order an EEG for me to have my brain activity checked out, because it couldn't hurt anyway. Christina and I thought it was probably a good idea, so we agreed. At that point, I was not keeping a journal yet, but I was having up to three or four of these in a day, and usually, at least one. He didn't seem nearly as concerned as we were at that point. He did have a diagnosis for me though. He told me that day, that he believed I was experiencing "visual migraines". He told me it is possible to have migraines without pain, and he believed, based on my symptoms, that was what was happening to me. He said the strange sensations and visual problems I was having were the auras that some people have at the beginning of the migraine. I wasn't really sold honestly, but who was I to question him. He was the neurologist after all, right? Maybe he was right? Also, I did sometimes have horrible headaches as a child, and my Mother does suffer from terrible migraines. Maybe it was genetic. He told me I should try a medication he had to offer. He thought it could help me out. He said it was not only a migraine medication, but it was an anticonvulsant. So, if I was having seizures, it may help, which made it a win-win. He thought it was a good fit. It made sense in my mind. It covered what I was thinking may be happening to me, and it covered his diagnosis. I figured I would give it a try. I didn't know what else to do, and sitting back having these episodes didn't feel like the answer. He also told me that day that I needed to "make sure I was enjoying myself." He wanted me to "go out and do things you love doing and have some fun." I felt as though he thought I was depressed or something, which I wasn't. I told him I was doing things I enjoyed frequently. He seemed to insinuate that he thought maybe these episodes were panic attacks, but didn't flat out say it. I knew they weren't. I was disappointed in that appointment, and was also losing faith in him as a doctor. I did however, have hope that this medication may help. Medication it was.

Chapter 3. Starting medication.

I was excited to start my new medication. I had some high hopes! Maybe these crazy episodes would finally go away! Due to the nature of the medication, you must go through a buildup phase. It takes some time. You cannot just jump to a full dose. You must start with a very small dose, and on a weekly basis, adjust your dosage, and eventually reach the target dose of medication. I remember, although thinking it was silly, feeling like a kid waiting for Christmas, hoping that by the time I hit my full dose, that these terrible episodes would pass. In the meantime, I tried to pay close attention to the number of episodes I had. That way, I would hopefully notice any change in the frequency of events I was having. I certainly didn't. I was pretty bummed out. I was trying not to let it get me down, but I won't be dishonest here, it got to me a little. It was frustrating. Slowly, one week at a time, I added one more pill to my daily routine of dosage, and still, no noticeable difference, at least in the aspect of what I was hoping for. I did, however, start to notice some side effects. One thing I started to notice, was my appetite seemed to decrease some, which was no big deal, I have a pretty big appetite, and it was not going to hurt me to eat a little less. I was a little happy about that one. Score one for the medication! I also did lose a little weight, which the doctor told me would likely happen, which seems obvious with the lack of appetite, and again, I didn't mind that! I was, after all, training to go back to the Department of Corrections, assuming all of it worked out. No complaints there. Then, I started noticing something I didn't like. I started struggling with mental clarity, focus and word finding. It seemed to get progressively worse as time went on. It got to the point where I felt embarrassed sometimes. I would forget words that you would never imagine forgetting. It seemed bizarre, and honestly, it made me uncomfortable. I knew that it was a possible side effect, but when it happens, it is weird. I would be mid-sentence, and just stop, because I just could not find the word. It would get to the point that I would have to ask for help sometimes to get through it, because I didn't know how to get out of it. For example. "Have you heard from?.... Uh...... umm... uh.... You know our uh..... you know.... Where is uh.... I'm sorry.. hang on... um....the person that gave birth to us?" "Mom." "Yeah, sorry, stupid medication." You can imagine how that can become embarrassing and hard to deal with in public. That slowly just started to become part of the program though. If the medication would have been working, I may not have minded so much honestly, but it wasn't. I was still having these episodes, and I still didn't really know what they were.

During this time, I had my first EEG done that the neurologist ordered for me. It didn't take too long to get in. I don't remember exactly how long, but it wasn't very long. My mother went with me down there. She is awesome. By this point, I felt like she was starting to have a little concern for me. I had told her what had been going on. Pretty much for the same reasons as I told Christina. I thought it would be wrong not to tell her at that point. I didn't want to burden her with worry, but I didn't want to keep her in the dark either. I am glad I told her. She has always kind of been a bit of a go to for counsel on subjects of things medical or complicated documents, etc. That's just kind of who she is. She is a helpful person who is always around to offer good advice. The type of EEG I had done that day was the type where they hook you up with all the electrodes (of course, all EEG's are) and then flash the lights at you to try and provoke a seizure, or seizure activity of any kind. They want you sleep deprived the day of the procedure, that way you can try and fall asleep during part of the test. If I recall correctly, the testing itself lasted around 30 minutes or so. It was honestly pretty cool. I quite enjoyed the lights. You have your eyes closed when they flash them at you because they are extremely bright. With your eyes closed, it's awesome. Or at least it was to me. It was fast paced blinking lights, but because of the way the flickering patterns changed, it made almost rotating shapes or something. Kind of hard to explain. It was cool though.

After some time, I got the results back of my EEG testing. It was normal. It showed no signs of seizure activity. Maybe the neurologist was right I guess, or so I thought. I knew that a normal EEG didn't mean you didn't have a seizure disorder, but I wasn't going to argue with him about it. I felt like I didn't have a leg to stand on, and I was not at all confident I was having seizures, it was just a guess that I had by reading some stuff off the internet anyway. This man went to school and became a neurologist. Who was I to argue with him? At least that was what I tried to tell myself at the time, and my fiancée. She always felt that there was something more to the problem then migraines, that was for sure, and deep down, so did I. I should have listened to my instincts and pressed the issue a little more, but again, hindsight is 20/20. I don't think, looking back now, I wanted them to be seizures either. It was much more comforting of a thought to think I was having migraines than seizures. Especially when I was wanting to go back into law enforcement. Maybe I went on allowing myself to accept that they were something that I knew they weren't, just so I could continue with the normalcy of life. Epilepsy is a hard pill to swallow, and I knew that long before I ever took it.

I was sure getting tired of the nonsense. I didn't know what to do though. I was pretty much at a dead end, or so it felt anyway. The medication had been in my system for a while now, and I just didn't really feel a noticeable difference. If it was making one, it wasn't drastic enough to be obvious, which to me, made it worthless. I had almost started getting used to the episodes. I was trying to find a way to both mentally and physically cope with them. If I knew I was going to have one, I made sure I was ready for it. I tried to make sure I was in a position where I couldn't get hurt and I wouldn't hurt anyone else. I had started telling more people what was going on. That way, if it happened, people knew. I was still working, so I let people at work know. I had friends at work looking out for me to kind of make sure things were alright. Like I had previously said though, usually, especially at the beginning, nobody really noticed them unless I was talking directly to them because if I was doing something, I would just continue to function as if nothing abnormal was happening. It was as if I were an android of some kind. As time progressed though, as they worsened, more and more people started to notice them. Especially one of my friends at work named Nick. He is a great man. He is the kind of person whom you can always have a deep genuine conversation with. Afterward, you will end up walking away feeling better about what you are working on, your situation, or even life in general. Nick is one of the people I had decided to talk to about my condition on a deep level. I did so because of the type of person he is. He gave me a lot of wisdom and insight. He helped me out a lot along the way. I have a lot of appreciation and admiration for him. He became very in tune with my episodes, even the very mild ones. He would sense them better than almost anyone. Better than anyone at work, that is for sure. He would look at me in the eyes after I had an episode, then kind of tilt his head and say, "you just had one, didn't you?" He never once asked when I didn't have one. He tuned me into things I didn't even know I was doing. I asked him after having one how he had known, and he told me I had been swaying, very slightly, back and forth while standing at the table I was working at. I had no idea that was something I had started doing during them. Nick gave me lots of good information, and I was later able to relay that information to doctors, who were then able to use that information to my benefit. So, now I would like to offer another piece of advice. Find the Nicks in your life. People who are around you daily, know you or your loved one's daily routine and mannerisms, and just talk with them. They are a fountain of knowledge. They can really help you out in ways you may not even realize at the time. People, just people in general are so important. You are going to need them. Listen to them. You never know who is going to be important to you and your loved ones during your journey. I have been through so much, and so many people have helped me in so many ways. Make sure you are receptive to the people who are there to offer real, true life knowledge, experience and wisdom. You may be surprised how useful some small comments end up being to you from a friend, someone like Nick, both medically and emotionally. Pieces of information about what you or your loved one may be doing during a seizure from people like Nick can be invaluable to doctors down the road. The life experiences they share with you, the friendly support and the compassion they may offer can do wonders for you or your loved ones. It is always easy to rely on those closest to us. Our family members, our closest friends, the people we spend all our free time with. It is important to remember though, people have many more connections than that. Do not dismiss them. Make sure you are open to the ones who are perceptive to you or your loved one's condition. They are out there, and they are an important part of your life. Not just in the cases with people whom have epilepsy, but in general, because people like Nick improve the lives of those around them, whether they are hindered by epilepsy or not.

    I had been at full dose for several months with little to no success. I was still having episodes on what seemed like a daily basis, at least on average. Sometimes, when I was lucky, I would go for a week, or a little more without one. That would feel great! I would start to wonder if it was working! Then, I would have several in a day. I would feel as though my body was "making up for it". It was so frustrating. I didn't know what to do. The episodes had pretty much leveled out. They were not getting any worse, but were not getting any better. I was still having visual distortions with almost all of them. Sometimes I would have the hallucinations, but not usually as drastic as the facial melting episode in the stereo shop. Usually the distortions would involve a "twisting" effect. It would look as though a section of my visual field would twist around itself. Almost like a "wormhole" looking effect that you might see in a sci-fi movie. It was certainly strange, but not nearly as bad as the melting face. That is for sure. Sometimes, all that would happen, visually, is I would experience a kind of visual "shaking" effect, almost as if I were standing on a loose platform that someone was using a jackhammer on. So, you can imagine how that type of vibration would affect your visual field. That seems to be the best way I can think to describe those types of experiences. I had also had another episode where I was riding my exercise bike and watching TV, when after the usual buildup sensations happened, the TV suddenly seemed to look three-dimensional. I certainly wish I had been keeping a journal during this period. I must say, that is when I had some of the most bizarre episodes of my journey, and some of the more important ones, as far as getting some of the best witness information. Like when I had the first one that Aldo ever witnessed.

Jimmy Golden. MY GOLDEN MIND, A JOURNEY THROUGH EPILEPSY AND BRAIN SURGERY

Aldo and I like to go and have lunch together whenever we are both off and get the chance. We usually just hang out, talk about riding motorcycles, what is going on with Supercross, maybe some current events in the world or just whatever happens to be on our minds that day. Aldo and I are very like-minded and see eye to eye on, well, everything really. As I said before, he is one of the people in the world of whom is nearest and dearest to me personally, and I confide in him as much as anyone I know. I trust him to no end. He is the kind of person who you know, no matter what, would always be there for you, and is only a phone call away, morning day or night. No matter what. He is full of wisdom, well beyond his years, and believe me, I have been fortunate that he is part of my life, for I have needed his wisdom and his help on many occasions, especially since epilepsy entered my life. I only hope one day, I can repay him for his kindness and generosity.

One day, Aldo and I went on one of our standard lunch runs. It was the usual routine. "Where do you want to go Junior?" "I don't know Junior? What about you?" That may sound confusing, but for years now, probably around ten,

Jimmy Golden. MY GOLDEN MIND, A JOURNEY THROUGH EPILEPSY AND BRAIN SURGERY

because of a long running joke that sort of got out of control, Aldo and I both call one another "Junior". It is so normal for us now, that it is a very rare circumstance that one of us slips up and accidentally calls the other by name. When it does happen, in a funny way, it makes us feel weird, and almost uncomfortable now. Almost like when a parent is mad at a child, and yells at them, calling them by their full name. "Jimmy Lee Golden! Get in here!" So, anyway, we usually quickly narrow our choices down between sushi or Mexican food. That day, we decided to go to one of our two go to Mexican food places to get some shrimp tostadas.

Before I knew it, I had an episode. I remember slowly regaining my cognition. "What was that? Are you okay Junior?" I remember the concerned look on Aldo's face. We were sitting in the Mexican food restaurant in our usual corner booth. I was feeling off, and a little out of it, but I was coming around. I had just experienced my first full blown episode in front of Aldo's face, while in conversation. "I just had one of those episodes I have been telling you about." I still vividly remember the look on his face. He asked again if I was okay, and I reassured him that I was. I was still feeling the aftermath effects, the tiredness and the slight confused feelings, but I felt like that one wasn't too bad. It wasn't super mild, but it certainly wasn't the face melting one. I was fine. No problem. I just needed a minute and I would be back to my usual self. Talking Supercross and whatever else came up in no time. He did look really concerned though, and Aldo is not unreasonable. Interesting, but unsettling. I honestly was not too concerned about it, because I still had a shred of hope that the medication would come around at some point. He was not so sure. He seemed more concerned about what happened than I was. I could understand his perspective though completely. If I watched my close friend, if I watched "junior" get stuck like I had just gotten stuck for a few seconds, unable to speak, just staring at me, almost like he was day dreaming, I would worry about him too. I understood where he was coming from. Definitely. He is a good man, and a good friend.

A few days had passed before I had thought to tell Christina what had happened, and that Aldo had witnessed one of my episodes during conversation. Even Christina hadn't witnessed one yet at that point. She had a wonderful idea. "You should talk to him about it Love. You should ask him what he saw from his perspective. See what it was like for him. See what he thinks. Maybe it was different for him than what you think." I don't know why I didn't think of that. That made perfect sense. I told her I would do that as soon as I saw him. At that point, after all, because of the doctor's diagnosis, I was still capable of going back to corrections, although, obviously, I really didn't think it was going to happen. I couldn't really make that kind of decision with something like that going on. Only if this stopped. I wouldn't go in with something like this happening to me. Not a chance. Too much at stake, both for myself, and other people. So, obviously, I really wanted them to stop. Not only because of the episodes in general, but they were influencing my potential career change at that point.

The following week, Aldo told me about some errands he needed to run, and some lunch to be had. He asked if I was interested in going along. I was, as usual. I typically have Fridays off, and sometimes, if he is lucky, he is "given" Friday off as well. Christina always works Friday, so, Aldo and I try to catch up if we are both free. We are usually able to find something to do. While we were out driving around, I remembered that I wanted to ask him about the episode. We had been talking about corrections. That is what put it in my mind. I wasn't thinking about it at first, but he mentioned that with what was going on with me, that he thought it was a little bit of risk to make that move. First and foremost, he was certainly right. Making a move like that with something of that nature going on with my health, when I already had a great job, would have been kind of crazy. Especially since I really do enjoy my job now anyway. I won't get into the pros and cons of one versus the other, it is just something I had been going through on a personal level I guess. Anyway, him saying that made me think about asking him about the episode at the restaurant. So, I did.

    I didn't realize it until I said it, but it not only felt a little awkward to ask for some reason, but I didn't quite know how to ask. "Hey Junior, I don't really know how to ask this, but can you explain to me what my episode last week was… like for you? I mean, how did I act, I guess?" It seems simple now that I am writing it, to just ask, but I remember when asking, it felt

Jimmy Golden. MY GOLDEN MIND, A JOURNEY THROUGH EPILEPSY AND BRAIN SURGERY

awkward for some reason. I think maybe it is because I am there when they happen, so to ask someone what I am doing, and how what I am doing makes them feel is just a strange concept for me to wrap my mind around. Or, at least it was back then, before I knew I had epilepsy. It has become easy over the past few years. I have become quite used to it now. I decided to tell him what it was like for me first. "I will tell you what it was like for me. I remember us talking. I started having those feelings I told you I have. I started feeling off, and could feel it coming a little, then all the sudden, I started having déjà vu. Suddenly I couldn't talk to you anymore. I felt stuck, like I couldn't do anything, and was just staring at you. I knew it was weird in my mind, but I couldn't do anything about it. I remember staring at you for a few seconds, and then, I felt that rush feeling come over me, then I could start talking again. I felt a little out of it, but I could function again."

It was his turn. I expected him to basically back up my version of events. That is not what happened though. What Aldo told me that day really made me nervous. I knew something was wrong already. The stereo shop incident, the pinwheel of color floating, spinning in front of my face. None of this stuff could be happening to me if something was not actually wrong, or at least that was what I was starting to think. Aldo, in my mind though, confirmed it for me, and made me realize it was really time to press the issue a little more with this doctor, or at least try. Try and see if I could. He hadn't been very responsive to my pressing yet. Aldo told me I was mid-sentence, and just shut off, like someone had hit an off switch. Then I just stared at him. At first, he just looked back at me, like you do when someone stops mid-sentence, maybe because they are thinking, or they lost their train of thought. Then my silence continued, and my staring continued. He said I had a weird look on my face. He said he asked if I was okay after a few seconds. I gave him no response or indication that I had heard him. I just stared, as if I were not there. He started to feel uncomfortable. He said he started to feel as though maybe he had offended me somehow. He asked again if I was okay. Still nothing. I just continued to sit, as if I were a shutdown android, not speaking, not moving, nothing. Perfectly still, silent, and staring at him. He asked again if I were okay. Nothing. He started to worry. Maybe it was something medical.

Jimmy Golden. MY GOLDEN MIND, A JOURNEY THROUGH EPILEPSY AND BRAIN SURGERY

A stroke maybe? He said he stood up and reached across the table, grabbed me by the shoulder and shook me. "Are you okay Junior!" Nothing. No response. I just stared. I was off. He didn't know what to do. He was thinking of what to do in his mind at that point, maybe it was time to do something. Then, suddenly, as though someone had turned the power to my brain back on, he said I picked back up, mid-sentence, right where I left off, as if nothing had happened. That is when he asked me "what was that Junior?" I was almost in shock. To me, this episode had lasted the span of a couple seconds. He told me it was probably closer to a minute long. I had zero memory of him attempting to talk to me at all, or him touching me. Yes, there was something seriously wrong with me, and it wasn't migraines. My brain was malfunctioning somehow. I was sure. In my mind, Aldo had just confirmed it. I may not be a doctor, but how else could that be? I was at a loss. Were they all like this, and I just didn't realize it? I had no idea.

I was getting fairly stressed out, at least on and off anyway. Sometimes I felt good, but sometimes, like after what Aldo told me, I felt pretty stressed out. Not too long after what

Jimmy Golden. MY GOLDEN MIND, A JOURNEY THROUGH EPILEPSY AND BRAIN SURGERY

Aldo told me, I was at home, alone one night, watching TV. Christina was out with a couple of her friends. I don't remember what I was watching or anything that night, but I remember I needed to go to the restroom. I paused the TV. I remember getting up, walking down the hall and to our master bedroom. Now, don't worry, I am not going to get into detail here, but I sat down on the toilet. I recall leaning forward a little and looking a little to the left and tilting my head. The image is still in my mind. I started feeling an episode coming on, but somehow, in a way I can't really explain, I felt like it seemed a little different to me. I didn't feel too well. I don't remember anything else. The next thing I do remember was waking up, in bed, the next morning, and feeling, well, beat up. I felt sore. My tongue was sore. Weird. Why was I in bed? I didn't remember going to bed... That seemed bizarre to me. Christina was sleeping next to me. I didn't want to bother her, so I just got up, and I went to the bathroom. I looked in the mirror. Under my eyes, I had what appeared to be a bunch of burst blood vessels. Really weird. Then I saw something else. I had a big, about the size of a quarter, dark red spot, which seemed to be kind of like a rug burn on the underside of my chin. I stuck my tongue out and looked at it in the mirror. The sides of it were bitten, bad. I had clamped down on it in my sleep for some reason. Again, weird. Then I noticed what I can't believe I didn't notice before. I was wearing all my clothes from the previous day! What was going on?! I woke Christina up. I asked her if I was in bed when she had returned home, and she had told me yes. She said that the TV was on pause, my cup was on the side table with my drink still in it (I am kind of a neat freak, I never leave anything out, that is a red flag), all the lights were on, and I was asleep, in bed, with all my clothes on. I told her I didn't remember going to bed, and what I had just discovered. We both wondered if maybe I had just suffered a tonic-clonic, or grand-mal type seizure.

I was still working. At that point, I was trying my best, without a journal, to loosely keep track of my episodes. On my worst day, I had ten. I contacted the neurologist and asked to schedule an appointment. I told his nurse, again, that I had new information that I needed to report to him, and that I needed to see him because I had been having some bad episodes. Again, she said she would call back and let me know. She did. This time, she told me, instead of seeing me, he wanted to just prescribe me a different medication over the phone. I, again, was shocked. What was going on with this doctor? Why did he never want to talk to me? I told her that I really wanted to talk to him, but I would consider it I guess. So, I did. Christina and I decided we were not thrilled with the medication choice he randomly threw out there, and we really needed to tell him what Aldo had told us, so we pressed the issue and ended up getting an appointment. At the appointment, I told him what happened, both with Aldo and with the strange night I had experienced. We assured him that Aldo is a trustworthy source of information, and that we were concerned with what he had told us. We really were wondering if I could be having complex partial seizures even though the EEG had been normal. He basically said that it is very unlikely for someone to have as many seizures as I would have to be having if were having them. He stood by his migraine diagnosis, but he would put me on the other medication that he wanted to prescribe over the phone to try it out if we would like. It was another type of anticonvulsant. He said it is a good medication, but I would have to have my blood work done from time to time to make sure the levels were correct in my system, and to make sure it was not causing any kind of kidney or liver problems. It also is known to cause weight gain. I was skeptical. So was Christina. I felt as though he was just trying to get rid of us. We didn't know what to do, or what to think. We considered the medication he wanted me to take, but we decided we really didn't like the side effect profile, especially when he didn't really give us good information for the reason he was prescribing it. I was torn because maybe it could help? At the same time though, we saw a lot of complaints about it. He didn't even seem to think I should be taking it. He was acting as though he was giving it to me just so I would leave him alone, and so he could show he did something. At least that was the impression we were getting from him. I don't know why, to this day, I hadn't already asked to change doctors honestly. I guess sometimes, in life, you just must learn things the hard way, and this was one of those times for me. I sometimes tend to give the benefit of the doubt, especially when it comes to professionals, even when the evidence suggests that I should do anything but. This situation, unfortunately, was one of the most significant examples of this that I have ever lived through in my life. I guess I just had to learn that lesson the hard way that time.

The first medication it was. The other one just seemed too extreme, especially without what seemed to be a real diagnosis. It was too much of a shot in the dark for us. Like throwing a dart in a pitch-black room, blind folded, after being spun around, and hoping for a bullseye. It wasn't too long before, again, after the incident with Aldo happened, that I started to get slightly used to my episodes. As used to them as one can get anyway. I don't think anyone ever really gets used to seizures after all. You just learn to tolerate them in your life. You learn to deal with them and accept them for what they are. You learn to live with them and expect them, be ready for them, or as ready as you can be anyway. It's not easy, but you don't have a choice, so you adapt, because you must, and you aren't going to roll up into a ball, and accept defeat. In a way, after a while, after something dark and difficult like epilepsy starts to take a grip on your life, even when it is undiagnosed, you start to learn from it. You learn about yourself. You learn what is most important to you in life, and you even learn valuable life lessons. You may not realize it, but it starts to change you. It starts to strengthen you, teach you to deal with adversity, teach you to overcome difficult situations and persevere. After some time goes by, you will see. If it is you that has it, you will see it in yourself. If it is a loved one, or someone you know, you will see it in them. Things that were difficult to deal with in life, are not so hard anymore. That person at work who used to eat away at you, who used to rent so much space in your head, suddenly is not so important. They don't mean so much, they become speed bumps instead of hills or mountains. Easy to navigate. A simple side note for you, your loved one or friend. In a way, that can be frustrating sometimes, but it can also be liberating. It is a matter of perspective. Teach yourself, or them to embrace it. That is important. Appreciate that in yourself, or in them. That doesn't mean that life is not difficult for us. It is. Epilepsy is, and will be difficult. Try and find and embrace what little bit of positivity you can find, and teach the others that are connected to the person with epilepsy to do the same. It helps with acceptance, and with creating an environment where everyone is informed and has a positive, rather than negative mindset over the situation, which is important.

The lack of progress, the lack of help from the neurologist, and the lack of evidence that the medication was making any noticeable difference, was making me question if I should even continue taking it at that point. People were noticing the side effects. It was getting harder at that point for me to deal with everything. I rather enjoyed my mental clarity after all. I am the kind of person whom, given the choice, will spend the evening watching the science channel to try and learn something about astrophysics, rather than indulging in mindless television, not that I have an issue with mindless TV. I have a few dramas I enjoy. The point is though, of course, the mental clarity issue was really a concern to me. The fogginess that I felt in my mind, the word finding issues, the feeling lost during simple tasks. It was taking a bit of a toll on me and was making me question if I should continue to take the medication. I was certainly losing hope that it was going to come around by that point.

Jimmy Golden. MY GOLDEN MIND, A JOURNEY THROUGH EPILEPSY AND BRAIN SURGERY

One day, I remember being in my bedroom. It must have been a Friday, because I was at home and Christina was at work. I recall needing to get something in the kitchen, so I headed in there. I walked in, walked to the sink, and tried to open one of those dummy panels under the sink that is not actually a drawer. I stood there for a few seconds trying to open it, repeatedly. Then I realized what I was doing and stopped. I thought to myself, "what am I doing!? I wondered why in the world I would try and open that. I know that thing doesn't open! I didn't just have an episode, I don't feel it. I feel as clear as I ever do. What was I looking for again? Why did I come in here? I forgot." Now, Of course, everyone walks from one side of the house to the other, and maybe forgets what they were doing from time to time, but trust me, this was different, and was not like me. I stood there, trying to get that thing open, absent mindedly. That is not me. I have never, in the entire time I have lived there, even thought about that panel. I know it is easy to blame medications on any little weird thing that may happen to yourself when you are on them, but lots of things like this had been happening to me since I started taking it. I was just foggy, unclear, not my normal, everything I do is for a reason and well thought out self. Everyone who knows me will understand that, I'm sure. It was a bummer, but I really didn't know what to do. I was thinking of trying to get off the medication. I just couldn't take the episodes and the side effects at the same time anymore. I at least wanted a clear mind. The neurologist had told me I didn't have to take it if I didn't want to. He had said I could try it and if I didn't like it, I could stop. I thought it was time to taper off. So, I researched it, found out how to do it, and I started to taper off. I was done.

Chapter 4. Let's see what happens.

The tapering of the medication was basically the same as going on it in the first place. Week by week, you take a small amount less and less. No big deal. I didn't feel any different, I didn't notice any changes in episode activity, I felt like I was making the right decision. I thought that after I got off, I would likely just go back to the neurologist eventually if the episodes didn't stop. I really didn't know what to do at that point anyway. Things obviously weren't working out. As I said before though, I was getting as used to the episodes as one could get, and was making due. I wasn't browbeaten or broken down over it. I was getting through them. I was keeping busy, I was working, and Christina and I were happy.

"Christina and I were happy". That is an important part of my story. I met Christina back in late 2006. Her Mother set us up. She works for the same company as me. It is a nice story. She works in an area that is a go to place for assistance, and to get things for the people whom do what I do for that company. I went to her area one day, and just like that, she asked me, "Jimmy, would you like to see a picture of my daughter?" I was surprised honestly, and a little caught off guard. I would have never anticipated anyone asking me that. I said, "yeah sure." I went back into her area and looked at a photograph of her daughter, and remember thinking she was beautiful. I told her "Wow, she is really pretty." The rest, as they say, is history.

Now back to where we were. During all this time, Christina had been quickly approaching the end of her Graduate program. We had always, without officially saying it, "planned on" getting engaged and married when she finished school. Even though I seemed to be "sick", somehow, she was starting to drop the little "hints" that it was getting to be time. Looking at, and starting to show me engagement rings and such. I knew it was about time. It had been, after all, almost a decade. If she hadn't been in school, we would have likely already been married, but we are the type of couple that takes things like that slow, and likes to have all their "ducks in a row", so to speak, before they do anything. I began giving some serious thought to getting her an engagement ring. I started talking to my friends at work. Nick, of course being one of them. I confided in him about my worry about being sick. He reassured me that someone whom had been with me for so long, stuck with me, loved me, and who had been by my side through so much, would continue to stick with me through illness, and I shouldn't concern myself with what was going on in that aspect. If anything, she would appreciate the gesture at that time. I decided he was right and it was time. I went for it. I found what I decided was the perfect ring, and I bought it for her one day when my Dad came out to visit. I had him drive for me, because at that time, naturally, I was avoiding driving until they figured out what was going on, although, the state hadn't pulled my license yet.

Jimmy Golden. MY GOLDEN MIND, A JOURNEY THROUGH EPILEPSY AND BRAIN SURGERY

I found a good hiding place in the closet for the ring. It was a motorcycle helmet box. She would never look there. She couldn't possibly care any less about motorcycle stuff. I put it there, tucked away, waiting to be presented to its first surprised face. Her father Ray. I wasn't sure when I was going to do it. I thought about it. I was trying to find a way to get him alone, which is usually easy, but for some reason, it was unusually hard after getting the ring. After a little while though, my chance came up. I was over with Christina, at her parent's house visiting, and he told me he was interested in running some errands and then going to my house to use my computer to down-load some music together. Perfect! I told him no problem. We were on our way!

Ray is more than "Christina's Dad." He is like a perfect combination of a good friend, and a second father to me. If I could design one in a computer system, I honestly couldn't come up with a better father-in-law than him. He will make marrying Christina all the better. We are often accused of "teaming up" together at family functions because we get along so well. I laugh at all his jokes, and his family makes fun of us for it. It is honest though. We just connect that way, we always have. I knew we would the day I met Christina on our first date, and I also met him, and he thanked me for taking her out "because, somebody has to…."

Ray was on my computer, I snuck off to my room, grabbed the helmet box down from my closet, and pulled out the beautiful diamond ring I had bought for her. I looked at it. I walked back into the office where he was. He was just about done. He asked if I was ready to go. I said, "I actually wanted to show you something first." I pulled the box out of my pocket and opened it. I showed it to him. He looked for a second and he took the box. He looked at me and said, "Are you going to ask her?" I replied, "yes, if it is okay with you of course." He looked at me and said "It's about time! It's only been, what, a decade!?" We both laughed, like we always do when we hang out together. Then he told me, "of course it is okay, you know we got your back, and that we love you." That really made me feel good. After everything I had been going through! Finally, a great day! We headed back to his house. We talked about it on the way there. I was excited! Awesome!

Now it was up to me. I just needed to figure out how to deal with these episodes so I could get healthy, find a solution and move on with my, no, with our life. That way, I can marry Christina and, well, live life as it comes. First though, I had to make sure I hid the fact that I had this secret now. No worries though. I wasn't concerned. I hid the ring back where it was. She would never find it. It was time to start formulating a proposal plan in my mind, while figuring out a way to get these episodes under control.

That night, Christina and I stayed up talking. Believe it or not, we talked about engagement rings a little. I, deceitfully, convinced her that I thought we should be waiting until we formally decide one way or the other about my potential career with corrections. I also convinced her we should wait until she is out of school, and has a job where she wants to be before we get engaged. I was kind of trying to throw her off a little, and it seemed to work wonderfully. I know it did, in fact, because I asked her later, after getting engaged. I felt a little bad, but I knew she would get over it when she got her ring. After all, I knew she wanted to be surprised. To think, all this time, she had a ring, just like she wanted, not 20 feet away sitting in a helmet box in the closet. We ended up falling asleep talking that night. It was the night of October 3rd, 2015.

A hour or so, I would venture to guess, after falling asleep, I woke up and needed to use the restroom. I got up, and I wandered in there. I came back out, washed up, and walked back to bed. On my way over, I looked at the clock. It was 11:30pm. I was tired, it couldn't have taken me longer than a few seconds to fall back asleep.

"Do you know where you are? Do you know what happened?" I was looking at someone I didn't know, in an unfamiliar setting. I tried to respond "no", but at first, I was so foggy minded and out of it. I was having a very difficult time functioning at all. I moved a little. The man told me, "try not to move too much, you are strapped down, but it is for your safety." Or something very similar to that. The original waking moments were very surreal and are unclear in my memory, but were, and are still there. He asked if I knew my name, I could mumble my name to him. I don't know why, but although I didn't know who he was at that point, I felt he was there to help. He asked again, "Do you know what happened?" I managed to reply that time. "No." He told me, "you had a seizure, you are in an ambulance, and you are on your way to the hospital right now. We are going to take care of you." At that point, I was clearing up some. My head was pounding. It wasn't like a normal headache though. It was deep. I imagined a tennis ball inside of my brain, and the pain was coming from the area where the tennis ball was only. He asked where I hurt. I told him my head, my tongue and my body was sore. I mumbled, but he understood. He told me I bit my tongue pretty good, my muscles were sore from convulsing, and that my head hurting was normal. Immediately, something dawned on me. I mumbled it out. "Who called 911?" "Your girlfriend" he replied. I remember thinking, "ah man, that sucks." The experiences of seeing inmates having tonic-clonic seizures taught me that seeing a loved one having one is something you never want to have happen to you. I felt bad for her instantly. "That sucks," I mumbled to him. He then started asking me a series of questions, presumably to gauge my state of mental functioning. He asked me what year it was, what month, what day of the week, the date, what I had done that day, how old I was, who the president was, why I was taking that medication I was taking, lots of things. Literally, the only thing I knew the answer to, was who the president was. What I found strange was, I knew what medication he was talking about, and I knew I should know why I was taking it, I just, for the life of me, could not figure it out. There I was, in an ambulance for having a seizure, the reason I was pretty sure I was taking that medication in the first place, and I couldn't remember why I was taking it. It was like the seizure had temporarily wiped out most of my memory. I had also forgotten what I had done that day, that I had asked Christina's father for permission to marry his daughter.

When I got to the hospital, they put me on strong medication to prevent me from having a second seizure. It made me tired. I got to have some visitors. Before I knew it, of course, Christina was there, and Ray and his wife Becky were there to support me, like always. It was good of them to come in the middle of the night like that. My family lived about an hour away at the time, and they showed up too. They had to pass visitor passes back and forth with Christina's parents to be able to come in and see me. I was so tired. Between the medication and the seizure, I was beat up and mentally exhausted. I was happy everyone was there though. It was nice to have the support. It made the experience much less of an emotional letdown. After some testing, and the hospital deciding I was not going to have another seizure, they allowed me to go home. I was ready to get out of there. I had to be helped in and out of the vehicle. I was just too messed up and worn down. The hospital had put me on a new medication and gave me a referral to see the neurologist. It was time to go back.

After that seizure, I went to work the following Monday. I told my supervisor what had happened. He was a different supervisor then the one who I had previously mentioned in this story. He told me "Oh, no, you need to take care of yourself man, you need to go report that to medical and get yourself checked out. Go see your neurologist and figure out what they say. Take a few days off, then see what happens from there. They aren't going to let you work right now. You need to get checked out and make sure you are okay. If the doctor releases you, then you can come in. Take care of yourself first man."

Completely different than my last boss. I was hesitant honestly. I didn't want to be off work, but I knew where he was coming from and I appreciated it. He is a good man. So, I went to medical. Like he said, they sent me home until I could see my doctor. I went and saw my PCP so I could tell him what was going on and get a work note to cover me until my neurologist appointment. I was officially off work at that point.

My next neurologist appointment came up. We went in. He, of course, saw what had happened. I will never forget that appointment. It changed the whole course of my journey. He basically told me that because of that seizure, it is obvious that the other event, the weird one where I didn't remember going to bed was likely also a tonic-clonic seizure, and all the other "episodes" I had been experiencing were, in fact, seizures. He was going to diagnose me with generalized seizures. We asked during the visit if we should do another EEG, but he basically told us that an EEG would just tell us that I was having seizures, and we already knew that, and that is if it even caught one. Also, I was on the new drug the hospital prescribed me, which was a good anti-convulsant, so I likely wouldn't have any seizure activity, so it probably wouldn't do any good anyway. I asked if this meant I had epilepsy. He said epilepsy basically means having two or more unprovoked seizures, so yes, I had epilepsy.

I was upset. We were upset. All the wasted time. He was going to leave me on the medication that the hospital had put me on. It had an awesome track record for seizure control, and had a decent side effect profile, at least as far as we were concerned. If I would have found a better neurologist from the start, maybe I could have avoided some of this. I was frustrated with myself. I should have listened to Christina from the start. She was right. The guy flat out missed the diagnosis. Oh well I guess, it was what it was. No sense in being upset over what was done. It was time to move forward. Now, I really felt like maybe we were on to something good! We had a real diagnosis, although it was one that was still a little unsettling for us, and we didn't really know what to think. My limited experience with epilepsy, after all, was with watching inmates in state prison have tonic-clonic seizures through the small window of a steel door, while waiting for backup to arrive so I could legally provide them with the assistance they needed in that high security building in which I worked. I still remember listening to the building alarm, wailing in the background, and watching frightened cell mates follow my instructions to help their cohabitant in need get through their difficult time. So, I couldn't help but wonder, "was that my future?" Without the prison cell, of course. After doing even more proper research, we were even more confident I had been put on a medication that had a good track record for stopping seizures, which at that point, we knew I was having for sure, obviously, because of the tonic-clonic.

It dawned on me. It was over. I was done. With that seizure, that trip to the hospital, that diagnosis, almost everything in my life had just changed. Although my life had really changed all those long months before, when I first started having my "episodes", I hadn't realized it yet. The thing is, it wasn't until that night, when I was rushed to the hospital, and I regained cognition, in pain, foggy minded in an ambulance, attempting to answer questions from the paramedic, that it really became official to me. I realized it the next day. My driver's license was now officially suspended, although I hadn't been driving anyway out of precaution, but now, it was official. The real tough pill for me to swallow though, was the thing that I had been dreading from the start, and it hit me. I had to call the California Department of Corrections. It was done, I was out. I felt like I did the day, many years before when I hesitantly turned in my badge. My heart was heavy the moment I realized it. It may seem funny to someone who has never been in that line of work, but I liked the prison environment. Don't get me wrong, I didn't love everything about corrections, but I miss many things about it. In the years since I have left, I purposely avoid driving by the prison to avoid stirring up old memories because, honestly, I just miss being there, and it is hard for me sometimes. As I said before, I love my job now, but law enforcement has always held a special place in my heart, and I guess, in a way, I still carry a torch for the Department of Corrections. That's life sometimes I guess. It looks as though the sounds of clashing keys banging around on my utility belt will live on in my memory only. No more walking the tiers of a maximum-security state penitentiary, proudly wearing a uniform that was earned through dedication and sweat. No more feeling the weight of the metal, golden badge hanging from my chest. No more smelling the smell of

Jimmy Golden. MY GOLDEN MIND, A JOURNEY THROUGH EPILEPSY AND BRAIN SURGERY

OC pepper spray in the air after breaking up yard fights and assaults, or hearing blaring building alarms as I run in, wondering what I am getting myself into this time. I will never again stop a suicide attempt and do my best to counsel a teary-eyed inmate, which after being in prison for over 20 years and realizing he no longer knew anyone in the outside world, had just found out that one week before his release date, his mother had passed away. I did my best to make him understand that his life was still worth living. I tried to explain that his loss didn't mean that he wouldn't survive outside of prison while living alone. It didn't mean that although after he was released, and he was initially homeless, with no money, and had that aching hole in his heart over the loss of his mother, that someone wouldn't find it in their heart to give a 50 something year old convict a second chance. It didn't mean that someone wouldn't provide him with a job, so he could try and earn an honest living, which is what he had promised his mother he would do throughout his stay in prison. It didn't mean that he should end his life. Instead, I told him, he should ask for help, because there are programs, and he should do what he thinks would make his mother proud. I still think about him until this day. I wonder what came of him. I truly hope I was able to provide him with what small amount of comfort an officer like myself could provide to a man in a situation like that. I hope he is out there somewhere, working, and living a rehabilitated and happy life.

Epilepsy stole those things from me. Then and there, with a simple diagnosis. I want to try and serve a purpose. Everyone does. I tried to help those in the prison system who wanted to get better, to get better. That is part of the goal of the California Department of Corrections. Rehabilitation. Now, of course, it was a law enforcement job. So those types of things are not your typical day on the job. Don't let me paint a false impression. I am not writing a prison book. I wrote about that aspect of the job, because it relates to the subject matter, and that is the portion that I miss as it relates to epilepsy. I also miss the excitement, the adrenaline, the "you never know what is going to happen daily" environment. My point of all of this is that sometimes, when having epilepsy, it gets difficult to not focus on, or to not get wrapped up in what you, or even the person you care about has lost due to epilepsy. Sometimes it is easier said than done, but try. Try and not focus on what has been lost. Try and focus on what you still have. Looking too much into what has been unfairly taken away will eat at you. No matter if you are the one with epilepsy, if it is someone you know, and you see the things it has taken away from them, or if by someone having epilepsy close to you, your life has become dramatically changed. Those things can and will be equally difficult for different types of people. It is important to understand that. The adjustment comes easier for some people than others, and that is okay. You will have to find ways to work through that. If that is the case though, and you are on the outside, try and remember, the person with epilepsy needs you, and they need you to understand what they are going through. Epilepsy is a two-way street though. It doesn't only take its toll on the person who has it. That is why you must always remember to communicate with others. No matter if you have it, or if you are a loved one or a friend of someone who does. Tell them how you are feeling and share things with those around you. Don't hold things about epilepsy in. Go online and read about things even. Reading about other people's experiences with similar issues that they may have gone through, may really make a difference for you or your loved one. Honestly, even read a poem, or simply just look up the word epilepsy on the internet and see what pops up. Search images. You may be surprised what simple, kind, warming and comforting things you might find, and what small group of words might comfort you or console you during one of your more difficult days or nights. Making it through the rough days and nights in one piece is another key to success.

So, seizures. It was settled. It felt kind of weird I guess. I didn't really know what to think. I didn't know if it made me feel better or worse. I was saddened because Corrections was done and over with, I was frustrated because the neurologist had missed the diagnosis for so long, and the fact that we thought it was seizures from the beginning only made it worse. I was looking forward to seeing what was going to happen with this new medication though. I had hope now. Again, I thought maybe we were getting somewhere. Maybe this was it.

Chapter 5. Time for a change.

We had decided. Even though I was on the new medication, I was going to request a new neurologist. It was time. I had been on the medication for a few weeks now, and was still having complex partials. It did seem to help though. I seemed to be having less of them. It was a start! I gave the neurology department a call and made the request. It was easy. It was so easy in fact that it made me a little more annoyed with myself for not doing it sooner. They scheduled an appointment to meet with my new neurologist soon after. I was still off work, which I didn't like, but there was no way that my company was going to accept me back, at that time anyway, and I knew it. It was okay, I understood. I was just honestly happy to be making some progress! Or at least that's how I was feeling. Trying to stay positive! Maybe this medication was going to work out and it would just take some time to really get it under control. Who knows? So, there was nothing to do but wait.

I am not good at sitting around and doing nothing, so I did a lot of research on epilepsy and complex partial seizures. I wanted to be prepared this time. I wanted to have questions and be somewhat informed about what I had when I met my new neurologist. I wasn't going to be as naive that time. That was my goal. So that was what I did. I found a lot of information of course. Epilepsy is certainly an interesting disorder. Intimidating. I just hoped I was going to get a good neurologist. I read that there are specialists called epileptologists who are neurologists that specialize in epilepsy. I thought to myself that maybe after everything I went through before, that was the way to go. Epilepsy is a complex thing. Even if the neurologist I got that time seemed like a good person, I thought someone who specialized in epilepsy would be ideal. Maybe we would ask. Christina agreed that it was a good idea.

Jimmy Golden. MY GOLDEN MIND, A JOURNEY THROUGH EPILEPSY AND BRAIN SURGERY

The day of the appointment, I was almost excited. I was really hoping I was moving forward. The first step at that office is to sit down with the neurologist's nurse. Then you have your vitals taken, then answer some questions and such. She seemed awesome. She told me I was going to love my new neurologist. I had a feeling she was right. I wasn't sure why, but maybe it was the confidence in her statement. Something told me though. We went in. We met my new neurologist. He asked about everything, although it was obvious he had already read my file and knew what was going on. I told him the types of things I had been experiencing. We explained some of the more concerning circumstances. He listened. He seemed like he cared about us. He was kind, gentle, friendly and his bedside manner was second to none. We loved him instantly. He told me I seemed to be having complex partial seizures. He said that what he would like to do is order an ambulatory EEG, which was a type of EEG that I would wear for an extended period, rather than for short time at the office like I had done before. I knew the answer before I asked, to a limited capacity because of my research, but I asked him if doing the EEG would tell him more than if I were "just having seizures". I told him the last neurologist that I had didn't order another one because he said it was unnecessary because we already knew I was having seizures. He seemed a bit shocked. He told me yes, it was a very useful tool since it will not only tell you if you have a seizure or seizure activity, but it also gives lots of information about the activity, including, but not limited to, where in the brain it is coming from. He also told me I would be able to wear the EEG home, would wear a belt with the recording device around my waist, and it would have the wires going up to the electrodes on my skull.

I had grown to like this neurologist so much in such a short period of time that I almost felt bad asking. I wanted to stick with the plan though. So, I decided to ask. "I don't mean this in any sort of disrespectful way, I value your professional opinion completely. I was wondering though, what would you think about me seeing an epileptologist?" His answer made me gain even more respect for him. He said that he is a neurologist, so he understands the mechanics of, and works with patients with epilepsy. The thing is though, it is a very complex disorder, his expertise in epilepsy is limited, and epileptologists are neurologists who specialize and devote their career to the study and treatment of epilepsy. He completely understood if I was interested in being referred to one, and he would be happy to send me to one. He wanted only the best for me. He asked if that was what I would like to do. I was shocked. He was an awesome person. We agreed. So, he referred me. He told me he knew of a great one within driving distance in the network, and told me her name. He assured me she was awesome. I was excited to meet her. He told me her office would contact me soon. He said that if I needed anything at all, to please let him know and that he would still help me with anything else I might need along the way. Most of the time, when someone has an epileptologist, they continue to have a primary neurologist. He is still my neurologist to this day. He is still just as wonderful.

It didn't take long to hear from the hospital where my epileptologist works. They set up an appointment for me. We were excited! Now I was really starting to feel as though things may be moving along. I wondered what she would think, I wondered how she would be. I hoped she was nice and friendly. My Dad took me to my first appointment. It was in Los Angeles.

Jimmy Golden. MY GOLDEN MIND, A JOURNEY THROUGH EPILEPSY AND BRAIN SURGERY

I was still having seizures. At that point I seemed to be having seizures around once a week on the new medication. It was helping, a little, but not enough. They were less drastic then they were when I was not medicated. That was nice but having one seizure a week was not okay with me if there was a possibility to do better. I had been off work for a while now. There was no way they would let me go back having weekly seizures. I was too much of a liability. My job is physical, so I can't blame them. I missed being at work. I was bummed out. I was having a hard time emotionally. I knew it was a combination of the diagnosis, the life changes, and the side effects of the medication. The seizure medications tend to cause you to feel down. I was having somewhat of a hard time adjusting. Especially with being at home, all day, every day, alone with nothing to do most of the time. There is only so much cleaning you can do. I paint sometimes. Acrylic or oil on canvas. That keeps me occupied, but it can be hard to find the motivation. Again, seems to be a side effect. But, it is what it is. I was having less seizures than I was, and I was going to see a epileptologist. I was trying to focus on the good. The glass was half full, not half empty.

"She is a very kind woman." That was the first thing I thought when I met my epileptologist. I liked her personality instantly. She introduced herself to my Father and I, and we talked some. She broke the ice in a nice way, it made the room very tension free. She then started asking questions. She asked about what had been going on. Just like my neurologist, it was obvious she had known prior to entering the room what had been happening to me. She asked me to explain, the best I could, what it was like when I have one of my "episodes." I believe, if I recall correctly, she called them episodes at the beginning. I know at first, she didn't call them seizures. So, I told her everything. I explained them the best I could. Just like my primary neurologist, she listened intently. She cared about what I was saying. She seemed to hang on to every word. She seemed as though she wanted to know, like everything I said mattered to her. It was as though if I could look through her eyes, I would see a recording machine and some sort of data analyzer. I could see it. What I was saying to her made sense. She knew what I was talking about. She was indeed an expert.

To hear her start talking. To hear her start working. It was incredible. The way she eloquently described everything to me made it all sound so easy to understand, and so non-frightening. Then, next, right away, she told me. Based on what I had just described to her, the same as I had described to everyone I had ever met with over my issues, she said she believed I was having complex partial seizures, and even predicted the area in my brain where they were originating. She explained everything in ways I could understand. She used models of the human brain to show where she predicted my seizures were coming from and explained why she believed that to be the case. It all made sense to me and my mechanically minded, yet malfunctioning brain. She was kind, gentle and understanding. She seemed to truly care about me and the situation I was in. I felt comfortable in her care. I felt at ease for the first time in a long time. She put my anguished, restless, darkened mind in a place where I could feel better, simply by speaking with me that day. She may not have known it, but that day was very consoling for my stressed mind. Like the other neurologist was going to do, she ordered an ambulatory EEG. Temporal lobe epilepsy is what she predicted. She also predicted where my seizure focal point was, or where my seizures were starting, based solely off speaking to me that day. I still tell people the story of meeting her. The analogy I like to use to describe the way I felt that day is, "it was as if I were trying to get information to build a rocket because the rocket I was building continued to fail. For information, I had been sent to see people who build model rockets they shoot off on the weekends. Sure, they may understand the mechanisms behind how rockets work, but they weren't helping. Then, one day, I got sent to NASA or JPL, and was sat in the room with a top rocket scientist, and she walked me through everything and told me exactly what was wrong and where the problem was coming from, right off the top, no problem."

I came back to the hospital shortly after my meeting with my epileptologist to be set up with my ambulatory EEG device. I had to wear it for about a week. I was excited. I was off work, I have a shaved head, and I wasn't doing much. It wouldn't interfere with anything, so I had no reason to worry about anything. EEGs don't hurt. They are just simply there. They can be a little annoying, and sometimes get itchy, especially after being on for that long of a period, but I was ready for the nuisance, that was for sure. I wanted to know what was going on! I was excited! Maybe myself and the doctors would get some good information. I just hoped, for the first time in my life, that I would have a seizure.

My dad drove me back to the hospital again to have the device put on. It was no big deal. They glue the electrodes on your head. You wear the recording portion around your waist on a belt. They also give you a medical video camera to carry around with you. The goal is to try and keep it pointed at you constantly, or as much as possible. That way, if you have a seizure, they can see what you are doing at the time. They want to see if you are smacking your lips, gripping your hands, posturing, etc. Anything like that really. The things someone does during their seizures can provide vital pieces of information to the medical team. Especially if you are going to head down the road toward brain surgery, which at that point, hadn't been mentioned to me yet. I used to do some of those things during my seizures. I would smack my lips sometimes, I would grip my left-hand open and closed, things of that nature. Again, great pieces of information for the medical team. Make sure you watch out for those subtle clues. They are windows into what is happening inside of you or your loved one's brain.

It wasn't long before a stranger was curious about my new headgear. My Dad and I had gone to a restaurant for some dinner. The waitress had asked if I was doing okay and wondered if I had had some sort of operation. I told her I was just fine, and I appreciated her asking. I told her I had epilepsy. I was having an EEG done to record my brain activity to see if they could catch a seizure, or some abnormal brain function to try and track down the area where the seizures were starting. It felt good to tell someone I didn't know what was going on. I decided then and there, I was not going to be quiet about my epilepsy. It's nothing to be ashamed of or to hide from people. I am going to do my best to let people know that people with epilepsy are normal. They are just like anyone else. They can be anyone. I am going to, by just being myself, by being someone with epilepsy who is not afraid to talk about it, spread epilepsy awareness so more people know about it. Leave my own little footprint on the world. Since epilepsy seems to have stolen law enforcement from me, maybe that's one of the differences I can make in the world. Just one of them.

After a couple of days, and while still wearing the EEG, Christina and I met up with her mother to go to one of our favorite restaurants to eat lunch. It was an extra special treat because that restaurant happens to be owned by two of our favorite people in the world, whom happen to be a couple of our nearest and dearest friends, Chris and Maira. After having some great Mexican food, we headed back toward Christina's parents. I was in the back seat. I remember one of their phones ringing. Next, the conversation they had seemed very familiar. I started feeling strange. I felt as though I had been through that exact situation already. They had already had the conversation I was hearing, and the phone call, it felt familiar in a way. The stop sign we pulled up to seemed to be the one I looked at last time the phone rang during that same conversation.... Oh yes, I was feeling it. It dawned on me. I was having a seizure, or at least I thought I might possibly be. I was not positive though, because it was very mild compared to the ones I usually had. I remember reaching down to my belt and trying to find and press the "mark" button on the recording device but having a hard time finding it. Pressing it tells the doctors that I felt something abnormal at, or around that time. It lets them know to really pay attention to that area in time, and, to know that if I did have a seizure, or seizure activity, that I am in tune with it. That ended up being the only "event" I had the entire time I wore the EEG. I was worried that I didn't have "anything". I was worried it was a false alarm because it wasn't that strong. It was nothing compared to what I have felt before. I worried, in a way, that I had a tonic-clonic only because I had tapered off my first medication, and it had only been a side effect from that, and that everything else could still just be something else, even though the neurologist and epileptologist now believed that they were seizures. As much as I didn't want to have epilepsy, I was more afraid of not knowing what was wrong.

After having the EEG removed, it took a few days or so to have it analyzed. I remember when my epileptologist called. I got out a piece of paper and pen and was ready to write. She told me that I was in tune with my body. The event I had marked was, in fact, a seizure. Not only that, but the EEG had recorded spikes, or irregular activity here and there during the week. It was coming from my right temporal lobe. Pretty much right above my right ear. Right temporal lobe epilepsy, intractable. That was the official diagnosis now. Intractable meaning that it is basically hard to control, and medication is not controlling the seizures. She was right. She had called it, right there, day one. All it took her was hearing me out that first day. She even properly predicted where the seizures were coming from. I was not surprised. After meeting her, after talking to her, I thought right away that she knew what she was doing. She was the textbook definition of expert. She wanted to schedule another appointment to talk about trying some different medication options and touch bases. The next thing she said started the next chapter in my journey. "Jimmy, with the type of epilepsy you have, you may be a candidate for surgical intervention, or brain surgery to stop your seizures. Would this be a route you would be interested in taking if you are found to be a candidate?"

Epilepsy had taken too much. I was frustrated, I was mad, I was burned out. I hadn't thought that question would be asked, but as soon as it was, I knew the answer. "Yes, I would be."

Jimmy Golden. MY GOLDEN MIND, A JOURNEY THROUGH EPILEPSY AND BRAIN SURGERY

Chapter 6. New plan, new hope.

Not long after speaking to my epileptologist on the phone, I was back in her office. She was fast. She didn't mess around. I really liked her, and she was growing on me more and more. We talked some more. She was good at comforting me. Every time I saw her, I always felt better. A little less on edge. Epilepsy had put me in a dark place. I won't lie. It has been hard on me, and it still can be. She has a way of making me feel less stressed about the whole situation. She had asked me how many "episodes" I had since the last time I had visited with her. I don't remember now, but I had kept track at the time. She informed me during that visit that it was time to start keeping a log of all my "episodes". She told me to log what day, the time, what happened during them, what they felt like and how I felt before and after. She also wanted me to log anything else I thought may be important, like what I had eaten, if I was tired, if I hadn't got much sleep the night before, or if I had consumed alcohol, which she recommended I didn't do at that point because it was a seizure trigger and would lower my seizure threshold, plus it didn't mix well with the medication. I told her I would do all of that. We also discussed medications. She asked me how I had been feeling emotionally. I told her I had been feeling kind of down. She told me it is normal to feel that way, with everything going on in my life, the changes, and it is also a side effect from the medications. I will remember forever what she said next. She asked me if I had any firearms in the house, and if so, she recommended I store them with a friend or family member. She informed me the medications are known to potentially cause suicidal thoughts and actions, and, after a seizure, in what is called the post-ictal state, I could go into a sort of auto pilot mode. I may wander around aimlessly, and do things without knowing what I am doing. I could potentially do anything while in that state that I know how to do while conscious. So, it is not a good idea to have guns in the house. That certainly made sense. All of it. I know firsthand, both how hard the medications can hit you, and how you can be perfectly fine one minute, then realize the next, you were just having a seizure, and were doing something you had no idea you were doing. Wandering aimlessly. I have had hundreds of seizures. I have had them virtually everywhere I normally go at this point. At work, at home, friend's houses, family's houses, while out walking, at the hospital, in cars, at the store, in parking lots, at an air show, at Disneyland, at a drag race in the grand stands, while exercising, while sleeping, while eating, the list goes on. I certainly valued all her advice, and she had plenty of it for me. I hung on to anything I could. I always brought my notebook so I could write down what she told me. If you or your loved one get involved with a doctor like this, cherish the bond you create. It will be important. It will make all the difference in the world. Trust me.

Although we had decided to pursue the surgery route, there was a lot to it. It was going to be a bit of a long road to find out if I was going to be a candidate. There was going to be quite a bit of testing. So, in the meantime, she said it would be best to experiment a little with medications to see if we can find something that works. As of then, I had been on two medications that had failed me, and really, it is best to make sure that there isn't one that works first. She told me that If two good anticonvulsants, especially the second one I was on, and still am on, failed, then the next step is to start combining a couple types together. She had told me that sometimes that is the trick with people who have a stubborn case of epilepsy. You just need to find the correct combination of medications. "So, while we begin the process of testing for neurosurgery, let's start seeing what we can do." It sounded like a good plan to me! I liked it.

She started me on a new medication, in combination with the one I was already on that the hospital had originally placed me on. She liked that medication too. She said it was one of the absolute best in her opinion. Awesome. In the meantime, she had put in a referral to set me up with a date to get me a spot in the EEG lab at the hospital for a six day stay for a video monitored EEG. She told me, this time, I would be admitted to the neurosurgery ward of the hospital, and would wear an EEG for approximately six days, would be confined to my room, asked to stay mostly in bed, and would be slowly, over the course of a couple days, tapered almost completely off seizure medication. Also, during this time, I would only be allowed to sleep a couple of hours a night. They would be basically trying to provoke my body into having seizures so they could record the activity. I would have a button on my bed railing so I could "mark the events" just as I did when I had the ambulatory EEG on. It was going to be almost a month out though. They don't have that many spots for that procedure, and it is in high demand. So, in the meantime, I would just have to see how the new medication would work out for me!

It didn't take long at all for me to decide that I didn't like the new medication. I felt very out of it. I was kind of loopy. My mind was slow and foggy. Not drunk, just slow. I had a difficult time functioning. Everything was hard to do. It was bizarre. I felt somewhat off balance, but not terribly. Kind of wobbly. I was off work, but the doctors encouraged me to continue and get exercise. They said absolutely no free weights. So, with that "restriction", I would go to the gym with Christina and just use the ellipticals and weight machines. I skipped most days at first while on that drug because I felt so "off", but I decided one day to go, not long into the trial. I remember Christina asking if I was sure, and I told her I was. She didn't seem to think it was a good idea. I didn't want to just sit at home if I didn't have to. I was already tired of being off work and sitting around all the time. So, we went.

When we got there, I remember I felt like everything seemed especially strange. I thought I would be fine though. I would just take it easy. I would just get a little light exercise and maybe it would make me feel better. As we entered the cardio area, we ended up seeing Christina's parents. That was a nice surprise. Ray noticed I wasn't feeling well. He asked if I was okay. We told him the new medication was just making me feel very slow and weird. He seemed a little concerned, but I didn't want to go home. I wanted to be out of the house for once. I felt as though I needed to move a little. I was mentally and emotionally burned out. I remember when getting on the machine, it seemed like it was more difficult than it should have been. Like it was technical, if that makes sense. I thought that was strange, but I let it go. We should have headed home right then and there.

We started working out. It felt good to get moving some. It made me feel better. The televisions at the gym have closed captioning on them so you can follow what is going on if you don't have headphones. I remember that I couldn't read it. I could see it, but I couldn't keep up. It was just too fast. My mind couldn't process the information fast enough to follow what was happening. It was kind of freaking me out a little, but I tried to tell myself I was just tired. I tried to focus. I tried, again and again, to read the captioning, and time after time, I would instantly fall behind. It was like trying to read movie credits in super-fast forward, but the TV was moving at normal speed, and I could see that. It was strange. It is hard to explain. We ended up getting off the equipment after a bit. I felt okay physically, but mentally I just felt so slow, like my brain activity had bad traffic. I don't know how else to explain it. Ray came up and talked to us again, and I seem to remember him telling us that we should go home. We ended up leaving. I believe they were leaving too.

Jimmy Golden. MY GOLDEN MIND, A JOURNEY THROUGH EPILEPSY AND BRAIN SURGERY

About half way home, my left hand started to shake, which is the hand that grasps when I have a seizure. I started to feel déjà vu. I started to feel a seizure coming. Then my hand started to shake more and more. I did something that got Christina's attention, although I don't recall what it was exactly. I was starting to have a seizure. It was different than my usual ones though, and I knew it. Then my whole body started to shake, but not shake in the way someone does when they are cold. It was more of a rocking back and forth of all my joints, and a jerking and twitching at the same time. I remember starting to clinch my teeth, breath hard, and kind of hit my head on the back of the head rest. Christina pulled over. I retained my consciousness. Weird. Then, it got worse. Slowly, progressively worse. Christina, because of the wisdom that my epileptologist had provided, had taken note to when it started. If it got to be too long, it became medically serious. My body convulsions were becoming on par with a tonic-clonic, but I maintained consciousness. It was starting to hurt, bad. My arms were beginning to beat against the door, the window, and the center console. My legs were kicking and pushing up and down on the floor board. My calves were burning, ankles, starting to take a beating. My neck was getting tired. My lower back and stomach muscles were burning from flexing back and forth from banging myself against the back rest. The best way I can think to describe the way it felt is this. It was like the feeling you get when lifting weights when you run out of strength. You are done. You are maxed out. Your muscles have given up and are on fire. They are in pain and your spotter is forced to help you finish. It was that pain but imagine it all over your body simultaneously. Now, imagine your brain refuses to take no for an answer from your muscles, and forces them to continue working out, through the strain, and somehow overpowers the muscle fatigue. I swear I felt as though I could feel the muscle fibers tearing throughout my body. Christina got out of the car and ran over to my door. She opened it because she was afraid I would break the window while convulsing and get hurt. By that point I was drooling. She didn't know what to do. I couldn't control my body. I can remember that much. I remember her asking what to do. She knew it had been too long. Even in the state of mind I was in during my seizure, I remember feeling the same way. I was being tortured by my own body. "C-c-c-c-c-all". That was all I could manage to get out. I wanted help, and I wanted it bad.

It continued for a couple more minutes, then slowly started to calm down, and as it was fading, I could hear the ambulance racing down the street. They pulled up to the front of her car, jumped out and came to help me. They ended up getting me out and onto the gurney. By the time it stopped, I had seized like that for over ten minutes. They decided they needed to take me to the hospital. I wasn't feeling well, as you could imagine. The paramedic talked to me after my breathing got back to normal. He asked me, "do you live on the west side of town? You look familiar." I told him I do. He replied "I think I responded to a call at your house a while back and took you to the hospital for the same thing. It has been a while, you must be doing pretty good with your epilepsy. Hang in there man." I thought that was nice of him. I thought he looked familiar too. I told him so. I told him that it must have been me, and that I appreciated it. I wished I wasn't having any seizures, but it could be worse, and him saying that made me remember that, right then and there, in an ambulance on the way to the hospital. He remembered me from the day I got permission to marry the love of my life.

After that seizure and hospital visit via ambulance, I let my epileptologist know what was going on. I told her how that medication was making me feel. She told me it was time to stop taking it, right away. That one, obviously, was not for me. So, I updated my log book, and I moved on. I held nothing against her of course. That was all part of the process.

So, it was time for my next trial. If I didn't try, I would never know. I was up for it. I was willing to have surgery, but I didn't see any reason not to try medications in the meantime. The way I saw it, I had epilepsy anyway. Most of my seizures were complex partials, but a few had generalized into tonic-clonics already. That seemed to mean I was at risk for that to happen at any time. That made me feel as though I might as well continue trying medications. "Big deal if I have another seizure due to side effects. At least I am trying everything I can to get better." At least that was the mind set I grew to have during the process. I was off work and wasn't driving anyway. I didn't care much at that point. I was having uncontrolled seizures already, and could not stop them from happening. I was in it for the end game, so to speak. I was focused. I just wanted to try and end my seizures if that was at all possible.

Before I knew it, I was on my next medication. That time, no craziness. So that was good. I didn't feel like a zombie. The main thing I noticed was that I felt a little off balance, but not terribly. I did also notice I gained some weight. I asked my epileptologist about it. She told me that it was not in the side effect profile for that medication, but it seemed like an abnormal amount of weight in an abnormal amount of time for me. I didn't really know what to think about that. I was still going to the gym and working out at least 4 days a week at that point. Nothing crazy, but who knows. Maybe it was me, maybe it was the medication. I guess I will never know for sure. Sometimes that is how it works. You can't know everything for sure in life. Where would the fun be in that? I would just have to work extra hard to try and stay reasonably healthy.

Jimmy Golden. MY GOLDEN MIND, A JOURNEY THROUGH EPILEPSY AND BRAIN SURGERY

The big day came! It was time for me to head to the hospital! I know it sounds funny to be excited to be admitted to the hospital for six days to try and have seizures, but I was. My parents had recently retired and moved out of state at the beginning of all of this. I was still in the dark about what was going on at that time. That was back when everything had just started happening, and my first neurologist made it seem like no big deal. Christina works full time, and at that point, she was still finishing up her master's degree, so we were fortunate enough to have my parents come down and help us out while I was in the hospital. We were very grateful. They ended up renting a hotel room about a block away from the hospital where families of people in the hospital seemed to frequently stay. We got there, I checked in, they brought us up to the neurology ward. They came in and got me all set up in my room. It didn't take long. Everyone there treated us like royalty. People there could not have been nicer to us. Before I knew it, I was hooked up, watching TV, waiting to have seizures, doing nothing. There really wasn't much too it honestly. They started tapering me off my medication, slowly, as I said, and that was about it. My epileptologist came in. That was the first time my mother had the pleasure of meeting her. The epileptologist was sick that day, so she was wearing a mask and gloves. I thought it was sweet that she was there at all.

If I remember correctly, I believe it was the second or third day before I felt something. I started feeling some funny feelings, the feelings I have become all too familiar with. I reached over and pressed the button. My Dad was the one in the room that time I believe. He didn't notice me acting weird or anything. I wasn't even sure it was anything. It was very mild. I was hoping it wasn't a false alarm. I feel a little like my Dad felt disappointed in himself for not noticing, but he certainly shouldn't have. Most people, after all, never even notice my substantial ones, even when I am right in front of their face, unless I am talking directly to them.

The nursing staff came in very frequently to check on me and see if I needed anything. They would also ask if I had experienced anything. I told them I had pressed the button and they seemed happy. I told them I didn't know though, it was mild. They seemed to have more faith in my judgement than I did. The next morning, I got a call on the phone from the epileptologist from home. She was reviewing my data and had saw that I had pressed my button. By this time, it was my fourth day, only two to go. They were keeping me awake 20 hours a day, while in bed. It was rough. I was tired. She told me that I was right. I had experienced a seizure when I pressed the button. Also, to my surprise, I had one in my sleep. I had no idea. That is great! She told me to keep it up. She really hadn't got what she wanted yet. She wanted to see a seizure where I grip with my hand, posture in some way, smack my lips or do something physical in general. Those things give another piece of evidence in support of the seizures focal point. This is especially true because the things I would often do during a seizure suggest to the focal point being on the right side of my brain, where they believed it to be due to the testing they had done so far. It would also help to make the case to the multidisciplinary epilepsy conference, whom make the decisions as to if surgery is a practical option.

Jimmy Golden. MY GOLDEN MIND, A JOURNEY THROUGH EPILEPSY AND BRAIN SURGERY

I was very tired. I just wanted to sleep. The EEG cap was becoming itchy. Don't get me wrong, it really isn't a miserable experience or anything, and it is worth every second because of the data they get, but I was ready for it to be over. On the fifth day, I felt another one. I pressed the button. This time I was pretty sure. It wasn't major though. No hallucinations, visual distortions or anything substantial like I have had. Just the feeling really. I just knew enough to press the event button. Sure enough, she called me later and told me the same thing. I was right again, and indeed had another. Awesome! Before the whole thing was done, I ended up having seven seizures, two of which were in my sleep. I caught all the ones when I was awake. The crazy thing is though, I was a little disappointed at first, because I believed that I hadn't really given her what she needed. All my seizures were very mild. No lip smacking, no posturing, no gripping of my hand. Just feelings. She had called me on the phone in the hospital every day to go over the progress of everything because she was ill and working from home. Much to my surprise, on the last day, she told me she had got what she needed. The last seizure was exactly what she was looking for.

"It was? What do you mean?" I didn't understand. She had told me the chewing movements and my gripping with my left hand during the seizure were exactly what she was hoping for. "I was doing that? I don't remember doing any of that. I just remember feeling my seizure feelings, so I pressed the button, then I just sat there, thinking I was sitting there doing nothing." She told me no, I had been doing exactly what she had hoped I would do, and wasn't surprised I didn't remember. It's normal to not remember things like that during a seizure. That was crazy. I mean, I know that happens of course, it has happened to me a ton of times. I had at least a few hundred seizures by that point, but it is still always weird to hear you don't remember something so simple when you feel like you clearly remember exactly what you were doing. This time, she had video evidence of it. Incredible. We were moving along now.

The next step of the process was to get a New MRI done. She told me that the MRI that the first neurologist had ordered was completely wrong for what she was looking for. It had to be done with "epilepsy protocols". That didn't take too long either. Aldo drove me down to have that done. People, and when I say people, I especially mean Christina, think I am weird because I kind of like having MRIs done. I find the noises the machines make to be quite soothing. I usually almost fall asleep by the time I am finished. So, I was looking forward to having the MRI done. The day we went down and I had it done, as per our standard procedure, we had lunch and conversation. It was good, as always. You must make the best out of everything. You must live every day for what it is, because when it comes down to it, life is nothing but a mega group of days. You can sit around and be upset that something like epilepsy has darkened that group, or you can do your best to enjoy them. I didn't have a seizure that day. I did, however, spend a day with Aldo, have a great lunch, and enjoyed the sound of the MRI machine and its clacking and swooshing magnets.

I had been waiting and wondering. I really, honestly expected to get MRI results that showed something. I was wrong. There was nothing. At first, I was let down. I was really starting to think brain surgery was the answer, and I thought to myself that a normal MRI result might, and probably did mean bad news. I talked to the epileptologist about it. She told me not to be concerned. She said it is common to get a "normal" result with my type of epilepsy, and it is still possible to be a candidate for brain surgery. All it means is that you don't have something, at least that the MRI can see at that level, in your brain, and there is no sclerosis of the tissue. She told me, in her opinion, it was a good thing. She said although it may make it more difficult to narrow down the spot in which the seizures are originating, it means that the brain material is not severely damaged in that area. She made me feel better, as she always did.

Jimmy Golden. MY GOLDEN MIND, A JOURNEY THROUGH EPILEPSY AND BRAIN SURGERY

Chapter 7. Moving along.

So, after the MRI came back negative, it was time for what was called my neuropsychological evaluation. I must say, this was another step of the process that I found interesting. I had to wait a little while for this appointment as well. I believe it was about a month. Christina took the day off work to take me to Los Angeles to have it done. The point of the evaluation is to test the overall functionality of your brain, cognitively, in different aspects and in different areas, to see how it is preforming, basically. This is my nonprofessional description of it, so please, look it up. It is very interesting. By doing this, they can, again, add another piece to the puzzle. If you are having issues in one area, and it happens to coincide with the area that they believe to be the area that the seizure activity is happening, then it helps back up their theory.

The test was very interesting and quite fun. The psychologist was outgoing, friendly and welcoming. We went to her office, but Christina had to stay in the waiting room. She worked on some school work because the entire process was going to take several hours, so she brought her stuff. The testing didn't take long at all to start. It began very, very simple, and it became progressively more difficult. I could tell it was designed to test different "areas of intelligence", if you will, or, different aspects of your brains functionality. There were memory sections, puzzles, trivia type questions, drawing and coordination type portions, and so on and so forth. Like I said, it was fun. Not at all intimidating. She made me feel very comfortable while there. She answered all questions I had, that she could of course. She explained everything thoroughly. I looked forward to hearing back from her after it was over, and after some time, I did. Over all, I did quite well, will a couple exceptions. My memory was not doing very well. My short-term memory

Jimmy Golden. MY GOLDEN MIND, A JOURNEY THROUGH EPILEPSY AND BRAIN SURGERY

particularly. My long term seemed to be okay. I was not surprised. I could tell during the test, but I knew anyway. I had been having a fairly difficult time with my memory since the beginning of all of this. During the test, it really hit me hard. Especially during one exercise she did with me. It made it obvious. To the point that she could tell that it made me feel nearly emotional. She comforted me that day during testing, she and told me not to worry about it. She told me it could be the medications, it could be caused from damage that the seizures are causing to my brain, or a combination of both. Either way, it wasn't my fault. She told me I would learn to work around it. She also told me that sometimes it gets better. Sometimes after surgery, people's memory can improve. She said I eventually may find new medications, my body may get used to the ones I am on, or I may be able just to stop using them one day because of surgery, then hopefully it will get better because I won't need them. She was a sweet woman indeed, and she did make me feel better about my slowly eroding memory.

Having epilepsy was really making me learn to appreciate people who are simply just kind. People who are friendly and care about others. People who are good to you because they can be. People who decide to be because it is the right thing to do, not because it makes their job easier. I was starting to meet more and more people like this through my journey, and they were making it easier than it would be otherwise. I really appreciated that. It makes a difference. I always do my best to make sure they know how I feel. Before we got off the phone the day my neuropsychologist called to give me my results, after she told me she had just sent the information to my epileptologist, I told her how much I appreciated all her kindness and how much her encouragement had meant to me. I thanked her for everything. One more step down. One step closer to surgery.

Shortly after, I heard from my epileptologist. She had received my results from the neuropsychologist. They seemed to be in line with what she would expect for having a seizure focal point in the area that she predicted mine to be. That was good news. Awesome! In my mind, it was more proof that she was great at her job. I really did enjoy hearing from her. Every time I did, she always seemed to make me feel better. She always asked me how I was feeling, asked me about the seizures I had experienced since we had last spoke, and asked how I was doing emotionally. She wanted to make sure I was doing well, and not just with seizure activity. I could tell she really cared about my well-being. I really had grown to appreciate her.

I told her I still noticed weight gain. I wondered if it really could be the medication, but she told me again that it was not a noted side effect. Maybe it was due to me being at home, not really being my usual, working and relatively active self. She was probably right. At that point though, I really was not a fan of the second medication I was on. I didn't really like the way it made me feel. I still felt slightly off balance on it. I also had noticed some slight blurred vision, which was one of the side effects of the medication. We had a good discussion about it over the phone during that phone visit. She asked me what I thought was best, which was refreshing. I was worried about trying something brand new, but I thought, other than the medication that I had the second seizure on that sent me to the hospital, this was the worst. She made what I thought was a good suggestion. She thought maybe it would be a good idea to try and combine the very first medication I had tried out, with the other medication that I was on, which the hospital had originally prescribed. Honestly, that was kind of what I had in mind. Although, it did make me feel a little foggy and forgetful. I felt more at ease taking that, then doing another trial run at something I had never tried. She thought that maybe the combination would be good. She said many of the other options were in the drug families of either the medication in which I wanted to get off, or the one that I seemed to have a possible seizure as a side effect from. So, going back on that original medication, and combining it with the medication that the hospital put me on, with the great track record, seemed like a great idea. We decided to go for it. Time to start the process of tapering up that medication again, and hoping it would make a difference. She also informed me that day of the next step of the process toward finding out if I was a neurosurgery candidate. A PET/CT scan.

Before I knew it, I was back at the hospital, ready for the next step. I had been gone through my tapering phase of my medication, and just around the same time as I finished, it was time for my PET/CT scan. Just like all the other steps so far, that one was no big deal. I found it interesting also. Nothing to be concerned about.

From my nonprofessional understanding, the PET/CT scan basically takes pictures of your brain while it is functioning. For the machine to do that, they must inject what they told me was a "radioactive tracer", which, of course they assured me is harmless. It didn't hurt at all. I believe they also injected some dye into my system. Which was also no big deal and was not painful. I believe there was a certain amount of time in which I was not supposed to eat before I arrived, but I do not recall the exact amount of time. It was not an extraordinarily long amount of time though to the best of my recollection. After they injected the "tracer", I remember being asked to relax for a while before the test started to give it a chance to circulate throughout my body. After the appropriate amount of time passed, I was escorted to the machine, where I was asked to lay on a table, on my back, and the table slid until my head was in the machine itself. Not my whole body, like when getting an MRI. The machine was much quieter than an MRI machine, and the scan seemed to last about 20 minutes or so. After I was done, they asked me to drink plenty of water to help flush the dye and the tracer, and I was free to go. No big deal at all. I was told I would hear from my epileptologist when she got the results, who would receive them from a radiologist who would read the scan images that would be produced by the machine. Great! I hoped they would find what they were looking for!

Christina and I had decided to go on a trip to a small town called Solvang. We wanted to have a little get away and have some fun. It was a chance to forget about what we were going through for a while, and just spend some time together. It was nice. I hadn't heard back about my results yet, but we would see. I was still having seizures with the new medication combination. I did feel a little better though. Out of all the medications I had taken, I liked that combination the best. I didn't feel as bad. I felt the most like myself. I didn't feel as much depersonalization between seizures. That feeling was something that had become part of my life since I acquired epilepsy. It was weird. That is one thing you, your loved one or friend may notice with epilepsy. At least it is something I had noticed. It was something, especially at the beginning when I was undiagnosed that really bothered me. It sometimes made me question myself, and even my sanity. It made things very difficult for me. I had a lot of depersonalization. While having a conversation one day with my older sister Jennifer, who I tend to have deep conversations with, I found the best way I could think of to describe these feelings. It is as if life is disconnected and not real for long periods of time, and even sometimes, constantly. When having these feelings, it's as if I could wake up and realize I had been dreaming everything that I had been living for a very long, but uncertain amount of time, and not be the least bit surprised. The analogy I realized described it best was, imagine you are watching television. You get really wrapped up in a show. You are deep into it. You are living with those characters; your life is one with theirs. You can almost smell the food they have on their kitchen table. You could almost add to their conversation, and they would respond to your statements. Then suddenly, the camera that is shooting the scene, for some reason, backs up, and it reveals that it is, in fact, the set of a TV show. You see the equipment, you see the people working off the set. You see the edges of the props, but still, the people continue acting. It draws you out of the false reality of the show. That is what it is like. When you have depersonalization, that is what real life feels like for you. It feels like a false reality. It is just some sort of a projection playing in front of your face, and you are waiting for the reveal, so you can witness the true reality come into perspective, so you can have your normalcy back. It doesn't come though. You are stuck in a perpetual state of waiting for the reveal, feeling distracted and perplexed. All the while, asking yourself if what you are experiencing is truly real, or if you are just imagining your illusion of disconnect. It is hard. It is exhausting. When you don't understand what is happening, it hurts. Epilepsy is more than seizures you see, if you have it, don't be afraid to talk about it. If you know someone who has it, don't be afraid to talk to them about it. They might need you, because there will be times when it is dark. Either way though, no matter who you are, always keep your eye on the light because that is how you find your way through and out of the darkness. It never lasts forever. Trust me, for I have been swallowed by the blackness of epilepsy many times before.

Jimmy Golden. MY GOLDEN MIND, A JOURNEY THROUGH EPILEPSY AND BRAIN SURGERY

I remember, while still in Solvang, and walking back to our hotel room after spending the day enjoying ourselves, walking around and sightseeing, I got an email from my epileptologist. I was nervous to read it. She had received the PET/CT scan results. I waited to get back to the room to read them. I hesitantly opened the email, worried that it would tell me something I may not want to know. At that point, after going through the amount of medications I had tried, my odds of finding one that would control my seizures were statistically much less than I was comfortable with, and the odds of a successful outcome from a "temporal lobectomy", which is what my brain surgery would be, would be much higher.

We went out for pizza that night! I was happy! One more step in the right direction! The PET/CT had lined up with all the other evidence so far. Awesome! I would have never imagined in a million years that I would be happy to hear that a PET/CT scan found an indication that there was some sort of issue with the workings and functionality of a section of my brain. I was though. Another box checked. One more T crossed and I dotted. I was starting to feel like I had a little forward momentum. Just maybe I had a chance after all. Just maybe I would be able to have a neurosurgeon remove the malfunctioning section of my brain one day, and hopefully stop these seizures. I did after all, have the type of epilepsy that seemed to be more likely to be operable, according to my own research. She also informed me of the next step. I needed to have another MRI. It was a different type though. It was going to be a 3 Tesla MRI. A more powerful and, because of that, more precise and better image providing MRI machine. More good news. I got to go hear the soothing and interesting sounds of my favorite medical equipment. Hey, the glass is half full, right?

Before I knew it, Aldo and I were off again. That time, because of the type of MRI machine required, we were headed to a different hospital to have the imaging taken. Aldo, being a reliable friend, like always, took the day off work to take me down there. As usual, we got some good lunch and had fun. It was funny though, because the day I had that MRI done, it was my birthday. It just worked out that way. I remember the staff at the hospital wishing me a happy birthday, which was nice of course. Everyone was very nice. That MRI lasted longer than the previous MRIs I had done in the past. I believe I fell completely asleep for a bit. I had contrast dye injected. It did not hurt or bother my system at all. No big deal. It was a good day. I was excited to hear the results. I hoped that they would find something in the area that would back up the PET/CT and all the other evidence that had been gathered.

When the results came in, I became worried. They were clean, just like all my other MRI results had been. They hadn't found anything abnormal. I wondered to myself if that was going to be bad for my case. Was it going to mean I would be ineligible for surgery? Were they not going to be able to "find the spot with enough certainty?" I spoke with My epileptologist about it. She had originally given me the results over email, so I asked to talk to her. She informed me that I should not be concerned with the results, and again, told me what she did last time I had negative results. "Just because they are negative doesn't mean you won't be able to have surgery." In fact, it was good in her perspective, in a way, for the reasons I had previously stated. My case was still looking good. They just needed to find other evidence. They already had some, they just needed to continue working. They already had evidence from multiple EEGs, a PET/CT, evidence from the neuropsychological evaluation and basically all the symptoms of temporal lobe epilepsy to go off of, such as my lip smacking, what I do with my hands, how my seizures feel, how they look, how I act, things of that nature. She reassured me. She made me feel better. Things were under control. It was a long complex process, and they just needed to really make sure everything was right. I could understand that. It was my brain after all. She did, however tell me that she was going to send my case to what was called the multidisciplinary epilepsy conference. They are a group made up of all types of neuro-professionals. They basically reviewed my case after it was submitted and were the ones who helped make the judgment call concerning me having neurosurgery. She would let me know what happened after it got reviewed. It was unlikely that they would go with surgery at that point, at least, that is how it seemed to me. They did have good evidence as to where the focal point was, but I was getting the idea that they were going to want a little more, and she thought the same thing.

It took a bit for her to get back to me because the conference only gathers once a month. So, I did my best to keep myself busy. I usually spent my time cleaning the house, going to eat sushi or Mexican food with Aldo on Fridays, painting paintings, text messaging friends, reading, researching epilepsy or catching up on vast amounts of television that I didn't need to be watching, but hey, why not right? I didn't have much else to do. During that time, we got an awesome little Yorkshire terrier and named him Oliver. I was hesitant at first. I love animals, but was not big on the idea of having a dog. I didn't really want to train one, pay for vet bills, and honestly, I remember all too well the heartache inflicted by all our old family dogs whom had become family members over the years. They became loved and cherished like a brother or a sister, then eventually, I remember having to say goodbye at the end. Rocky, Ranger, Thunder, Cayenne, Tobey, Dolly, Bonnie, Bailey, Comet… Christina hadn't lived through that yet, until recently when her mother's beloved Hercules passed. It was a sad day for all of us. He was a little Maltese with a big attitude, but a lot of personality, and he brought a lot of joy to the whole family. He is much better off now though, because he had fallen very ill, and we all felt very sorry for him. It was time, and ultimately, the decision was placed on the family. I was proud of them that night for doing the right thing, and putting his needs before their emotional interests. I think Christina understands why I hesitated to get a dog now, but honestly, Oliver has brought a lot of happiness to my life, and of course, hers as well. He has helped me tremendously through this journey. He has made my days at home feel much less lonely, and his constant happiness to see me makes me feel good about myself, and I love him for it. It turns out, she was right about getting our little Oliver, just like she was right about that first neurologist.

The multidisciplinary epilepsy conference had met. They seemed to think she was headed in the right direction, but they needed more evidence before they would move forward with surgery. At least that is what I got out of the conversation. One thing was certain and crystal clear though, more testing. I figured that would be the outcome. I was ready for it. I had done some homework and figured I knew what was next, and I was right. It was time for a MEG scan. I was ready. The sooner the better. She told me I would hear from someone soon.

It took a little time to hear from the hospital that was going to perform the MEG scan for me. It was going to take some time to get it done as well. I was let down a little. It was what it was though. There are not many MEG machines in the country, and they are very important, so it is not easy to get a date. I just had to wait. Back to TV and hanging out with Oliver!

During that time, Christina graduated from college with her master's degree! Hooray! I was so proud! Awesome! We had a party for her at the house, it was nice. She had worked hard and it had paid off, after all that time! It is important to try and not get so wrapped up in the craziness that you forget to live not only your life, but engage with your loved ones. I know it can be hard sometimes, believe me. It can beat you down. I was 30 years old at the time, my fiancée just graduated college, everyone was over at the house, we had great food, everyone was having fun, having a few drinks, letting loose! Not me though. I can't drink alcohol, it is a seizure trigger, and it reacts with my medications. It's not worth the risk to me. I didn't want to end up on the floor or in an ambulance and ruin the party. I ended up having a complex partial that night anyway. It wasn't too bad though. Some people noticed, but hey, no ambulance, no hospital, it could have been worse. I took it as a win! I am lucky because I am one of the people with epilepsy who is surrounded with people whom, for the most part, understand what I am dealing with as much as one can be expected to understand, and don't try and peer pressure me into drinking, or give me a hard time about things. They don't make me feel bad about having seizures, they don't think I am possessed like some people do, they are understanding. They aren't overly sensitive about the topic. I am surrounded by good people. I talk about it with those who ask, and I tell them anything and everything they want to know about it. I think that is important, and I personally believe that is one of the keys to having successful relationships with those close to you in your inner circle when you or someone you know, care about or love has epilepsy. Openness and honesty about the subject. Teach them about it. If I have a seizure in front of people that know me, I am confident, almost anyone I know would be fine, and would make the right decisions, regardless of what kind of seizure I had. Imagine a world where everyone was that way. Awareness is another key to success.

Chapter 8. This is starting to look good.

Finally, it was a long wait, but it was time for my MEG scan! Again, I was starting to feel bad about it. On second thought, no, I felt bad about it a while ago. Aldo was taking another day off work to take me. That time it was even worse. It was about a four-hour drive to get to the hospital where the MEG machine was located. Aldo really is the man! I don't know what I would do without the guy. I hope I can repay him someday, somehow, without me having to drive him to crazy amounts of his own medical tests, of course. I certainly wouldn't wish this nonsense on him.

Jimmy Golden. MY GOLDEN MIND, A JOURNEY THROUGH EPILEPSY AND BRAIN SURGERY

We left very early that day because he thought it was a good idea, just in case. I felt bad doing that because it just meant he had to get up earlier to take me. "Come on junior, it's fine, I get up super early for work anyway, don't worry about it! You never know Junior, you don't want to miss your appointment because of something stupid like traffic." He was right, especially on the freeway we were going to have to take, but I still felt bad. So, I hesitantly agreed.

It was a good thing we left when we did. There ended up being a fire on the side of the freeway and we got stuck in bad traffic. We ended up making it to the place right on time! I couldn't believe it! Aldo basically saved the day! I was so glad! Who knows how far back that would have set me.

We went in and I did the paperwork, it wasn't much. The people were very friendly, just like everywhere else. They explained some stuff about the MEG, which, I recommend you look up, because the science behind it is incredible. I won't bother trying to explain it, because it is way beyond me. They set me up. The cap they put on me was just like an EEG cap. They glue the electrodes on. After that portion, they use a device and trace the outside of your head, in between the electrodes and all around your face and jaw, almost as if drawing on you with a pen. That sends a signal of some sort to a computer I guess, and it maps your skull out in the system. It felt kind of good. No pain or anything whatsoever. They asked me some questions about my seizures. I'm not sure if it was part of the test or if they were just curious. After all the set up was complete, they brought me into the room with the actual MEG machine, which looks like a giant helmet that you sit in a chair under. You must take off any kind of metal before going in the room. Metal will interfere with the readings. The room itself shields the machine from outside interference of any kind. It really is interesting. After you are in the chair, it raises up and your head goes into the machine and you just relax for the duration of the test. It is very quiet. Toward the end of the test, they put a very mild stimulation pad on my wrist that made it twitch so that my fingers would move. It caused brain activity to happen that they wanted to read. Not painful at all. It kind of felt good. The whole test was quite pleasant. I enjoyed the experience because they explained things to me which I found fascinating.

It took quite a while to get the results back from the MEG. I was warned that may happen. The problem is that those machines are extraordinarily expensive so there are very few of them in the country. So, if someone gets into a traumatic accident, or is found to have some sort of life threatening ailment and may need brain surgery right away, they use the MEG to map out the brain for the surgeon, or to locate the brain damage. These cases, of course get priority and bump cases like mine. Then, when they move forward, they also get their data analyzed first, which is very time consuming. The scan itself lasted, I believe around twenty minutes, but the data is analyzed by the millisecond, rather than the second. They were not just looking for seizures, they were looking for, in my case, "temporal lobe spikes", which are very short bursts of irregular brain activity, or short blips of discharge that happen on a very small and short scale. They look for the source of the "spikes" on the MEG results with pin point accuracy. With those results, they hoped they could obtain a more clear and detailed perspective of where my seizure focal point was. So, you can see why it takes so much time to comb through the results of these tests. On top of the time it takes alone, if you are bumped by someone who's life may be hanging in the balance, it may certainly take even longer, which, of course, I wouldn't mind at all. Before I left that day, the woman at the front desk told me I was supposed to go to their sister campus to get another 3 Tesla MRI with the epilepsy protocols that their doctor prefers. When having an MEG, they use MRI images to build a bit of a 3-D picture of sorts. I was not aware of this at the time. I called my insurance company and they told me to go right ahead. I felt bad, now Aldo had to drive me there too. He didn't mind. Looked like lunch and dinner that day! He is a true friend. I sure have had a lot of MRIs for a 30-year-old. I had an ACL reconstruction surgery, which required two follow up surgeries a couple years prior and had to have a couple MRIs for that as well. No wonder I liked the sounds of them!

After some time, some television, quite a few walks around the neighborhood to keep busy, and a lot of quality time with Oliver, the results were in. It was good news! The MEG results found exactly what they were looking for! Temporal lobe spikes in the exact area that lined up with the EEG results from the hospital, the ambulatory EEG results, the neuropsychological results and the PET/CT results. All of that on top of the general evidence that they had received from me that was collected from the observations of my family, my friends like Aldo, Nick and also myself. We were really onto something!

I talked to my epileptologist on the phone. She basically congratulated me at that point. I could hear it in her voice, she seemed like we were really on our way! I was excited. At that point, I was really hoping for surgery. I was tired of having seizures. At my age, having later onset epilepsy, it really hit me hard. I was struggling with it. I was struggling to stay positive. Losing my driver's license was difficult. I am not your "watch football on Sunday, go out at night, drink and party" kind of guy. I grew up riding motocross. I have raced motocross, I raced motocross sidecars for a while, I used to ride street bikes (crotch rockets and Harley Davidsons), I used to competitively drag race a street bike within a racing organization, I used to own a 1965 Nova race car and competitively race that at tracks all over southern California with a group of other racers, I have been sky diving several times, I have been bungee jumping, and like I said before, I was planning on going back into Law enforcement before all of this. Seizures devastated my lifestyle completely. I didn't know what to do when I heard the diagnosis of epilepsy. I knew what it meant though. I don't mean literally. Of course, I literally knew what it meant. I have witnessed the darkness of epilepsy through a piece of thick, state owned prison glass several times before. I have tried to communicate with inmates in post-ictal states, and not been able to get through to them because they were too confused. I knew epilepsy meant seizures. I also knew it meant that my lifestyle had just completely changed. My driver's license was now a state ID, my truck was no more than a tool for friends and family to borrow, my beautiful motorcycle and bicycles had become dust collectors, corrections had become a memory, not a future. All of that is why, when my epileptologist asked me if I would be willing to have a surgeon open my skull one day, and try and repair my malfunctioning brain, I instantly responded "yes". I didn't have to think about it. There was only one answer for me. If there was a chance for me, I was ready, willing and enthusiastically going to take it.

Jimmy Golden. MY GOLDEN MIND, A JOURNEY THROUGH EPILEPSY AND BRAIN SURGERY

Chapter 9. One last thing.

The moment of truth was coming. I only had one test left to find out if I would be deemed a surgical candidate. I was told it would be an interesting one, and that it was called the "WADA test". It was going to be the most invasive test of the entire process. I did my best, as always, to research it. It turned out, during the procedure, they were going to insert a catheter into an artery in my groin area and run an angiogram up through my body and to the back of my brain. They would then inject an anesthetic, and one hemisphere at a time, they would shut down my brain. The cognitive function of one hemisphere at a time would be tested, while the other was essentially nonfunctional.

They would also inject a dye, and take images, therefore mapping out the pathways of the arteries inside my brain. That way, if I did end up having surgery, the surgeon would basically have a map of what was going on in my brain, as far as arteries were concerned. They wanted to be sure I didn't have any abnormal arteries that were, for lack of better words, out of place, which can apparently sometimes be the case. I was getting to learn all kinds of interesting things about the human brain.

Based on the reading I was doing about the WADA, people either said it was very interesting and enjoyed it, or they thought it was uncomfortable and really disliked the experience. I didn't find anyone really complaining about pain, which was comforting, it was more of the strangeness that people didn't seem to care for. I was curious and just thought to myself, "it is what it is, if it is uncomfortable, at least it won't last forever I guess. I must have it done. I need it for the study, and it does sound a little interesting." I am honestly not one to be afraid of doctors, dentists, or anything like that. So, I was not too worried. It was going to be a while before I could get in though. I had some time to kill. It is a specialty test, and they only do it in one room of the hospital, or so it seemed. I had to wait for it to become available.

An annual racing event was coming up in Las Vegas. It was called the Street Car Super Nationals. I used to compete in it in my Nova and on my ZX-14 street bike back when I drag raced motorcycles. I ended up getting to go to that race with my friend Ron because I had so much down time while waiting for the call for my WADA test. So, the wait wasn't so bad after all. Awesome, I found another glass half full in the situation. He used to race in it also, but, at the time, he was going up there solely as a crew chief, always selflessly helping run his sister Lori's S-10, ¼ mile, 10 second drag racing pickup truck. He always makes the long haul in his motor home, brings all his tools and equipment to make life easier, more fun, comfortable, and tolerable for anyone and everyone who decides to involve themselves in all the drag racing events she races in. Ron has an "open motorhome door" policy of sorts. Come one come all. We pack in like sardines if that's what it takes for us to all indulge in the racing action and good times! That is who Ron is. He gives and gives, and we sure all have a lot of fun. Ron was the friend who had introduced me to all the racing in the first place. Ron is much older than I am. He is honestly more of a friend/father figure kind of role in my life. I have often told people he has done as much, if not more for me than anyone I have ever met in my life who is not in my immediate family. Ron helped my father and I build that 1965 Nova race car I used to own. I, when I say "helped", really mean he was the brains of the build, and the one who did most of the main work. We were more like lost helpers, my Dad and me. My Dad and I have been working on cars forever, but Ron is just on a whole different level, and race cars are a whole different game than street cars. When we brought home that Nova, he told us to "bring that thing on over" and it ended up staying in his garage for who knows how many months, getting nearly fully rebuilt. Kudos to his lovely wife Kelly for putting up with that. She is wonderful. Ron took me to many doctor's appointments while on my journey through epilepsy. Throughout this story so far, they had just been some of the less pertinent ones, so I hadn't mentioned them. Ron had not only driven me around for doctor's appointments like Aldo did, but, like Aldo, Ron would always find ways to get me out of the house. He was good at making sure I didn't spend too much time alone. He would call and check on me from work, on his weekends, after he knew I had appointments, when he was going to run errands, or when he was going to work on his lake house. He would often come pick me up, so we could spend some time together. He knew I needed time away from the solitude. He is a great man, and I will never forget all the things he, Aldo, and everyone else did for me during this journey. Chris and Maira, the ones who own the restaurant, would do the same. They have picked me up and brought me to breakfast. Chris has taken me to Los Angeles on runs for restaurant orders numerous times. During several of those runs, I had seizures, which never deterred him from taking me again. My parents and my sisters, obviously. My little sister Brittany just sent me a text message last night with a picture of a flower, in epilepsy purple, that she wants to get tattooed on her arm for me. I played it cool, but I was at a loss for words. Ray, it goes without saying. He would do anything for me, I know it, and I for him, and he knows it. Christina. She stuck by me. It has been hard, she could have left, but she didn't. She has so much going for her. She is young, beautiful, has a master's degree, is a professional, makes great money, the works. Yet, here she is, sticking it out, and I will be forever grateful. The list goes on and on. These people, I was, and still am at a loss. You never really understand how important people really are, until you go through something like this.

While sitting at home, eagerly awaiting the WADA test, I decided to do something that I had been wanting to do for quite some time. I figured I had the free time. Things were not quite as hectic, and Christina was at work, so I could do it without anyone knowing. I didn't want to tell anyone I was going to do what I was planning to do. I was a little embarrassed. I knew that my odds of being successful were slim, and in my mind, I thought possibly even none. Now, this book is about trying to help people. I am writing it because when I was going through what I am describing, I was unsuccessful when trying to find something that described a journey through epilepsy and brain surgery in a first-person account. I searched for a book like I am writing because I wanted to understand what it would be like. I wanted to get a better idea of what I was going to go through. I wanted to know someone else's take on the pain, all the darkness, all the suffering, the testing, the issues and the questions that may arise. I wanted to hear someone else's perspective who had been through all the craziness already because I thought it may help, even if everything about their situation was not precisely the same. I wanted to know what kind of small pieces of advice they may have to help me get through the times that lie ahead. I had a difficult time finding anything like that, and ultimately, I failed. That is why I am here, to try and help others who may be on a similar journey. Help loved ones of people with epilepsy, or people whom they know. Hopefully spread more epilepsy awareness. That being said, what I am about to share is personal, and I am not trying to press any kind of political beliefs or agenda. I want that to be clear. Everyone has their own opinions, and that is what makes people individuals. Now, while waiting to have my WADA test, waiting to find out if I would be a surgical candidate, I decided to do something I had wanted to do for a long time. I was running out of time to do the task that I had been wanting to accomplish. I wanted to take the chance to write a letter to the President of the United States. Barack Obama. I knew the odds were long.

Jimmy Golden. MY GOLDEN MIND, A JOURNEY THROUGH EPILEPSY AND BRAIN SURGERY

Chances were, it would never make it to his desk. I thought to myself, "you know what, you should just take the chance. Go for it. You never know what could happen. Stop being so negative. Just write him the letter and tell him your story. Tell him what you want to tell him." My story about epilepsy isn't all I wanted to tell Barack Obama. I had thought for a while, if I ever had the pleasure of meeting him, I would tell him a little story, and I would also tell him something else. I decided to go for it, even though the odds were long indeed. Here is what I wrote.

Dear Mr. President.

I will be honest sir, it took a little time, but you completely won me over during the past eight years. I thought I would share my story of why, and how, and with the hope that you will get a chance to read it and see the unexpected positive impact your presidency has made on my life.

I grew up in the small town of Phelan, CA in a republican household. I went through school and did well, got great grades, but never had a particular interest in any further education beyond high school, nor did I pay any attention to politics. I went on to work for ------------, then left to become a California state Correctional Peace Officer in 2008 when you became president.

I didn't pay much attention to the election. I was a new Correctional Officer at the time and was very busy and had little understanding of politics now that I am looking back. I still remember the night you were elected. I was working at the California state prison in ---------- known as ----------. I was on the night shift working in ADSEG or administrative segregation as the only officer on the floor. I had heard that you had won the election, and to be honest, although I didn't pay too much attention to the election, I was neither happy, nor particularly upset. I will remember that night for the rest of my life. I went out for a security check, and while walking section C of the upper tier, a soft spoken older African American Crip inmate stopped me and said, "excuse me Officer Golden, do you happen to know who won the election?". I was hesitant to tell him. I didn't really know the protocol for situations like that, but I felt like he had the right to know, and I thought to myself "what harm could it do?", so after a few moments, I said "yes sir, Obama won." He just looked at me for a second and thanked me and I went on my way. I would say about thirty seconds later I heard him start yelling out in excitement.... and I knew I was in for a long night. The building erupted in cheers... People banging on doors. It was a night to remember. I also remember, my last count before morning, I noticed lots of inmates had packed their belongings. I asked one of them what they were doing, and they told me that now that you were in office, they were getting out. I just shook my head and went home.

About fourteen months after joining the Department of Corrections, I received multiple layoff warning notices due to the state's financial crisis. I was devastated. I had left a job with -------------- to become a correctional officer, and when they found out, they offered me a pay raise to come back. In fear of losing my job, and the window of opportunity to get back into ---------------, I went back to ---------------. Giving up my Badge was devastating, but I felt like it was the right thing to do for financial security.

Jimmy Golden. MY GOLDEN MIND, A JOURNEY THROUGH EPILEPSY AND BRAIN SURGERY

During all this time, I lived with my roommate, who unlike me, was more political and left leaning. During our time together, we had many discussions that really shaped my views of politics and opened my eyes about the world. I specifically remember one conversation about me being a republican and my thoughts about you. He had asked me if I considered myself a democrat, republican or something else. I told him proudly that I was a republican. He simply asked why. I realized at that moment for the first time in my life that I had no clue. I could not believe it. I was so embarrassed. It seemed so simple, and yet it had never crossed my mind. I just grew up in a republican household, and I guess I just embarrassingly enough, blindly identified as a republican (although, come to find out, my views are typically the exact opposite of a republican). You had happened to be on TV that night. I mentioned that I didn't particularly care for you.... He again simply asked why. Again, I didn't have an answer. I had no idea. I knew that you being elected caused my housing unit to become more difficult to manage at work, but obviously that wasn't your fault. I really knew nothing about you other than you wanting to reform healthcare, which I understood

Jimmy Golden. MY GOLDEN MIND, A JOURNEY THROUGH EPILEPSY AND BRAIN SURGERY

nothing about. I really felt speechless. That conversation was, for lack of better words, life changing for me. I became interested in politics after that. I now care what happens in the world. I follow politics. I wonder how I went so long knowing so little about what is going on in the world. Now, I myself use similar simple questions with people who seem to be in the same state of mind I used to be in myself. My way of paying forward what my friend did for me. Its seems to work on others as well.

A Little over two years ago, I started considering going back to the Department of Corrections. My girlfriend (who is now my Fiancée) was getting close to finishing her master degree in speech and language disorders (which she since has). My job at ------------ is a specialty kind of job and so if I stay with the company, we will have to live here indefinitely. So, since I had decided to propose to her, I was going to go back to corrections so we could live anywhere in the state, and as a speech and language pathologist, she can find a job anywhere, and her parents would eventually go with us and hopefully become happy grandparents. During the hiring process for corrections, suddenly I started having strange "spells" that I couldn't quite describe to my doctor, and I was sent to the neurologist. He diagnosed them as "painless migraine auras". He told me that they were harmless and not to worry about them. Myself and my girlfriend were a little more concerned than he was because they seemed more drastic than he seemed to accept. We worried that I was having seizures.

I went on with the hiring process. The doctor cleared me and I was approved even with the "spells" and was waiting for an academy date. I was going to be picked up as a "permissive reinstatement" at my old prison by the warden because I had already been an officer and my process was expedited. Everything seemed great, other than the "spells". They worried me, but I trusted the Doctor and went about my business and tried not to worry my girlfriend. I Bought my girlfriend her engagement ring and decided to ask her before I went off to the academy. I officially asked her father while we were spending some time together, and of course, he was excited. Her and I had been together for almost ten years. It was past due.

Jimmy Golden. MY GOLDEN MIND, A JOURNEY THROUGH EPILEPSY AND BRAIN SURGERY

That very night, her and I fell asleep talking. I was excited, but hid it from her because I was going to wait and ask her at Disneyland around her upcoming birthday. It is, after all, her favorite place in the world. Later that night, I woke up in an ambulance, confused, and I had no idea what had happened. The paramedic started asking me a series of questions I still remember. He asked what day it was, I had no idea. He asked what month it was, I had no idea. He asked what I did that day, I had no clue. He asked why I take a medication I take, and I could not remember. He asked me who the president was " Barack Obama". I remembered that one! I had a tonic clonic seizure in my sleep in our bed next to her. I woke her up having convulsions before I stopped breathing for a minute. My "spells", as it turns out, were in fact a combination of simple and complex partial seizures. As of now, I have had hundreds of them. I have epilepsy. I had to cancel my plans to become a correctional officer again, and I am now on social security and am currently waiting on one final test, called a WADA test on Dec. 5th at the - ------------- Medical Center in Los Angeles CA. If I pass that, I will be scheduled to have brain surgery to remove a large

Jimmy Golden. MY GOLDEN MIND, A JOURNEY THROUGH EPILEPSY AND BRAIN SURGERY

section of my right temporal lobe because my epilepsy is considered intractable and cannot be controlled by medication. If I don't make it back to work by the two-year mark, I will be medically terminated. At that point, I will have to get health care with a "preexisting condition". So, you can see how important the ACA is to us just in that one aspect. Our wedding is currently on hold until we can get all of this squared away. My fiancée is strong though, and she sticks with me. She looks up to you and your wife, as do I. We watch your and Michelle's speeches and are inspired. The affordable care act is so important to people in situations like ours. I just wanted to take the time to thank you. I know that chances are, I will never have the opportunity to shake your hand or thank you in person. So, I wanted to take the opportunity to express my thanks the only way I know how. Thank you for the past eight years and for the things you have done to help my family and the family's in situations like mine. It seems by watching you and your family on TV that you are strong people, but I can only imagine that the negativity must get difficult from time to time. I hope that the letters of thanks from people like myself and others that take a moment to express our gratitude, make the sacrifices you and your family have made worthwhile and serve as a reminder of what you stand up for daily. You are a people's president, and the people who really sit down and listen know that. Again, thank you President Obama, I wish you luck on your post presidential endeavors.

sincerely,

Jimmy Golden

I walked over to my mail box, and I dropped it in. That was it. All I could do now is hold on to a sliver of hope that it would make an impression on the staff that tirelessly read all the letters that pour into the white house daily, by the thousands. I hoped, that just maybe, it would strike a chord with the people who would read it at some point. I had an idea how it worked. If that first person who read it selected it, they would pass it on. It would then go to another pile of selected letters to be read by another staff member, who then had to narrow it down into another pile. That staff member chose another small group of letters out of that vast pile, and placed them on one final person's desk. That final person had the difficult task of reading through, and narrowing down the large pile of letters selected, who had made it that far, and choose the ten letters in which that person believed would "speak" to president Barack Obama in some way. President Obama read ten letters a day from citizens of the United States, and I decided, however long the odds, to try and become one of them. If nothing else, it was my chance to try and express my thanks for protecting people like myself with preexisting conditions, who may lose their employment due to no fault of their own, and would find it difficult to gain insurance without the new law his presidency had propelled into action. I felt more at ease because of this. At least with all that was happening with me, I would be able to get insurance. I would not be able to get denied. Another glass half full. That was the way I was trying to see the situation. Looking for the positive. After putting the letter in the mail, I basically let it go. I never told a single soul. The way I looked at it was hey, if I even received a card from the White House one day saying thank you for writing, I would be excited! That would be awesome. Even better yet, it would be great if it was signed by some sort of staff member or something! I didn't dare dream that big though. I tried to let it go. I must be honest though, I always held on to a shred of hope. Just maybe, maybe I would get some sort of reply from a staff member. Who knows.

It was time for the WADA! Boy, was I ready! I had scoured the internet looking for videos. I had only really found one. It was old. It was interesting though. It gave me an idea of what to expect. I had searched discussion boards about the test. I had a hard time finding a whole lot about the subject matter. I did find some though. It seemed some people had great experiences. Some people really enjoyed it. I even found one person who said they would do it again if they could. I thought that was interesting. I also found a person who was not much of a fan. Most people seemed to be neutral. I was starting to get the impression that when the hemisphere of your brain shuts down that is non-dominant, you may end up feeling, and acting the ways you do when you have a complex partial seizure. I don't remember exactly what made me think that, I just remember getting that impression by the way people were talking on the discussion boards.

Jimmy Golden. MY GOLDEN MIND, A JOURNEY THROUGH EPILEPSY AND BRAIN SURGERY

Ray, Christina's Dad, drove me down that day. He had taken the day off work for me. It was a two-part test. I had to go down on two separate days. The first day was to get you familiar with the test and the process. They wanted you to know what to expect. They have you watch a video, and they talk to the person that will be with you on the day of the actual procedure. It didn't take too long. It was a Friday so we got to hang out and get some dinner after. I was glad Ray could take me. Aldo had been taking too much time off already, so I really didn't want to ask him, and Ray had gladly volunteered. We went back the following Monday for the actual WADA. It was great because Ray got a four-day weekend out of it! I didn't have to feel quite as bad about him taking the time off. I was going to have to stay in the hospital for observation for a while to make sure I didn't bleed from the hole where they ran the angiogram into the artery in my leg, or act funny after the testing was complete. The recovery time was scheduled for several hours.

When I got there, I was admitted to the hospital because of the type of procedure it is. It is considered invasive, so they are cautious. They treated me wonderfully though. Everyone was great. I had no problems. We got in quickly, and they prepped me for the procedure. They had me put on a gown, hospital socks and a head sock. Next, they brought me into the prepping station. They had to shave and prep my groin area because the catheter they put in goes in the artery at the very top of your thigh, right where it connects to your groin. After I was all prepped, they had me say goodbye to Ray and they carted me away to the room where they would perform the WADA test. I remember thinking it was interesting looking in there. Everyone introduced themselves. There was a psychologist to do the cognitive function testing, a doctor for the angiogram portion (I can't remember what they are called unfortunately), an epileptologist (not my primary because she had gotten sick, but we did not want to postpone the testing), and a few other medical professionals to assist.

While the helping professionals were setting up, the artery doctor was explaining to me how they use that room to do surgeries to repair stroke victims. It was cool. He was a nice man and it kept me nice and calm. I appreciated that. Once everything was set up, it was time to place the catheter. They opened my gown, sterilized the area, which is a little embarrassing, but otherwise just fine. He gave me a small shot to numb the area. It did not hurt at all. Just a tiny pinch on my upper thigh. After a minute or two, they went ahead and started inserting the catheter into the artery. Again, no big deal. It just kind of felt like someone pushing on the top of your thigh. Nothing to worry about. Before I knew it, it was in. Cool, we were good to go! It was time to start the angiogram portion!

I could feel a slight dragging feeling at the site of the catheter, which didn't hurt at all, it was just a little sensation. I suppose it was the feeling of the angiogram tube sliding through the catheter tube. Other than that, I could not feel a thing. I could tell they were watching the screens to see where in my vascular system the tube was heading. Eventually, after not long at all, I felt a slight warming sensation in my face. I thought to myself "I wonder if they accidently injected something?" I said, "my face feels warm, is that okay?" The guy running the operation looked at me and said, "did you just say something?" I replied "Yeah, my face is warm, is that okay?" He said "yes, we have injected the dye into your brain, try not to move okay? Be very still from now on. Don't talk anymore." I remembered thinking to myself that he probably should have told me before he injected the dye in the first place. I then thought, maybe he did, and I just either didn't hear him, or I forgot. Who knows. They had been really on top of everything else. That was for sure. Oops!

I looked over, with just my eyes, and I could see a slight view of one of the monitors where the continues x-ray cameras put up images. It was the image of the dye running through my brain. It looked incredible! I remember thinking, "so I have a brain after all! Wait until I tell Christina!"

Within a couple minutes, the epileptologist and the psychologist came to me. I was laying on my back on the table. They had me strapped down, head and everything, but it wasn't bad. It wasn't tight. One came up to each side of my head. They told me it was time to start the test. Awesome! I was ready! Last test! Let's get this show on the road!

The psychologist told me a phrase. She said, "Johnny swims in the swimming pool." She said she wanted me to repeat the phrase to her. So, I did. She told me she wanted me to try and remember the phrase. Then she showed me a piece of paper with a red circle on it and asked me to identify what it was. So, I told her it was a red circle. She told me she would ask me to do the same thing later. She then showed me a flashlight and asked me to tell her what it was, and I did. She told me to remember she had showed me that object. Then she explained she would show me various items throughout the test after the drug was administered, tell me statements and ask me to remember them, show me colors, shapes, objects and so on. After the test, she would ask me to remember the things I was shown and would be asked to do my best to remember all sorts of things from while one hemisphere was shut down. She would show me objects and ask if I had seen them or not, show me colors and ask if I had seen them or not, ask me to repeat the original statement, and so on and so forth. It seemed simple enough. I was ready.

It was time. They told the helpers to administer the drug. When doing so, the epileptologist had me cross my arms on my chest, then she put her pointer finger and middle fingers together on her right hand. She asked me to squeeze them as hard as I could, and while doing so, to simply start counting out loud until she told me to stop. I grabbed her fingers like she asked and started to squeeze. I was a little afraid I would hurt her fingers honestly. At first, I held back. She looked at me with kind eyes and said, "squeeze my fingers as hard as you can Jimmy, you aren't going to hurt me, trust me." So, I did. Her fingers popped in my hand. I guess she was right though, she didn't even flinch. I began counting out loud. "One, two, three, four, five, six." I counted well into the thirties before she stopped me. She stopped the test. There was something wrong. She needed to check something. The angiogram had moved ever so slightly, and by doing so, was not allowing the medication to reach my brain properly. So, I was perfectly normal. I felt perfectly normal too. I had thought I felt normal. I kind of laughed to myself and thought "man, I thought I was killing this test! Ha-ha! Guess not! I thought the drugs were just not really effecting my non-dominant side much!" I had read that feeling normal when the side that is non-dominant is under anesthesia is common, but also sometimes, you may feel a little strange, so I was curious what would happen to me.

Jimmy Golden. MY GOLDEN MIND, A JOURNEY THROUGH EPILEPSY AND BRAIN SURGERY

They made the necessary adjustment. The psychologist made sure I remembered the original statement. I told her again "Johnny swims in the swimming pool". She said we were good to go. She told them to administer the drug again. She again, had me cross my arms and squeeze her fingers as hard as I could, same as before. The test began.

Due to the fact they were putting what was projected to be my non-dominant side to sleep first, my right hemisphere, she put her fingers in my left hand. They did that so I could squeeze using muscles controlled by the right side of my brain, which would be impacted by the drug during the test. In the human body, the muscles are controlled by the side of the brain opposite to the side of the body they are on. If you move your left hand, the electrical activity that made that movement happen, came from the right side of your brain. That is why the information from people in your life like friends, family members, coworkers, outside observers, the Nicks in your life, the people who care enough to notice and pay attention to what is happening to you or your loved one is so important. The fact that I consistently did things, like grip my left hand, or grab my shirt with my left hand during seizures was a big clue that the seizure focal point, or starting point was in my right hemisphere. It was another piece to the puzzle. I owe thanks to all the people who took the time and cared enough to notice things like that, and reported what happened to me while I was cognitively absent during all my seizures. It helped build my case for the multidisciplinary epilepsy conferences to come.

"One, two, three, four, five, six, seven, eight, nine, ten," I was laying on my back, counting. Clear as a blue summer sky. I felt as if nothing was happening. Squeezing her fingers, still feeling a little bad about it. Then about when I get to twenty, she slapped my hand a little and said, "keep squeezing Jimmy", I said "I am, sorry." I thought maybe my grip loosened a little. I was worried I was squeezing too tight, but I was also getting a little tired from squeezing so long. So, I clamped down. I continued to count. She said something to the psychologist. "He is about a" and said a number in which I don't remember. I didn't understand it at the time. I was confused, but I didn't think much of it. I was concentrating on counting and squeezing. I figured it had to do with the medication entering my body. She slapped my hand again. Slightly of course, just a friendly tap. "keep squeezing Jimmy, come on Jimmy, keep squeezing for me." I told her I was. I kind of thought it was funny. I don't have a light grip. When I tested for the Department of Corrections, I passed the grip test, on the grip machine, while adjusting my grip and kind of testing to see how it felt, to see what kind of resistance the device had. I hadn't even given it an effort yet. And now this epileptologist is tapping on my hand telling me I wasn't squeezing her fingers hard enough, when I was trying hard to squeeze. I thought it was kind of funny. Again, she tapped me "keep squeezing Jimmy, come on, keep going!" I almost thought for a second she was messing with me. She again told the Psychologist another number "he is at a", then she told me to stop counting.

The epileptologist asked me how I was feeling. I told her I felt perfectly normal. I was ready for her to tell me the catheter had slipped again. She told me "You have a strong brain!" I said "really, is the drug in there?" She told me the drug was indeed in my brain and I was being affected by it. I was shocked. I had no idea. I felt perfectly normal. I would have never guessed. She asked me the statement we had talked about. "Johnny swims in the swimming pool." She asked what object she had showed me. "A flashlight." She asked about the shape and color. "A red circle." It was honestly like talking to someone any other day. I felt like they had done nothing to me at all.

Next, she started telling me little statements and showing me pictures, shapes, colors, objects and such. Then, after a little bit of that. They gave me time for the medication to wear off. It was that easy. No big deal at all. I didn't know any different because I felt so normal anyway. I had no indication anything was different about me anyway. After the time had passed for the medication to clear my brain, they returned to ask me the series of questions to see what I remembered about the experience while under the effects of the medication. They asked all about the things they had showed me and talked about. I would honestly be surprised if I got much or anything wrong. It was easy to remember most, if not all of what happened during that part of the test. I hear sometimes that is not always the case though, even during successful WADA tests. They told me I did great and it was time for the second part of the test. She asked if

Jimmy Golden. MY GOLDEN MIND, A JOURNEY THROUGH EPILEPSY AND BRAIN SURGERY

I had any questions before we moved on. I told her I did. I wanted to know if my grip strength was effected much by the drug, because I really didn't notice much of a change. "oooooh yes Jimmy, that was why I was tapping on your hand and telling you to keep squeezing. You weren't gripping my hand at all anymore. The left side of your body was paralyzed from the medication, that is how we know it is working, especially when we are doing the non-dominant side. That is why we have you squeeze. You were not able to squeeze at all; your brain only thinks it is still squeezing at that point." I was blown away! My brain was tricked into thinking I was struggling and my muscles were growing fatigued from squeezing this poor epileptologists hand. I couldn't believe it! That test really was bizarre!

    I remember thinking it was time for the interesting part. I knew that shutting down what was likely to be my dominant side was going to be bizarre based on the research I had done on my own. I do recommend self-education during your battle with epilepsy, whether you are the one inflicted with it, a family member, a friend or just someone interested. Knowledge is power.

"Here we go!" I thought to myself. I began to squeeze, that time with my right hand. "One, two, three, fou…" That was it. I was not even able to get through the word four. I was done. The medication had completely interfered with the workings of my brain. In a way, it felt a little like it does when I have a complex partial. I felt a little déjà vu like and strange. Next, my memory became foggy, but I still recall clinching my eyes shut and bursting out in laughter. I could not control it. Nothing felt funny to me, I just laughed uncontrollably. I had moved my hands and was shaking in some way. I do remember that. I couldn't stop laughing. I remember the epileptologist telling me to "stop it". I couldn't though. I believe I eventually stopped laughing. They eventually began the testing and started saying things to me, and showing things to me. Since my eyes were clinched shut, one of the doctors would have to use her fingers to pry them open and the other would hold the objects or cards in front of my face and show them to me. They would ask me what they were and I would remember attempting to answer. I was basically useless. It was so strange! It was one of, if not the most bizarre experience of my life! I remember at one point them showing me a picture of a bicycle. I knew it was a bicycle, and when they asked what it was, I managed to get a word out. I tried to say bicycle, but the wrong word came out. I don't remember what it was, but it was the completely wrong word, and I knew it, but there was nothing I could do about it. It was crazy!

After they finished, they walked away. They gave me the time required so that the medication could dissipate. After a while I felt back to my old self. The epileptologist and psychologist returned and began asking questions about what I remembered. I did my best to answer the questions. I did remember some things they showed me, and a couple things they said for sure. A couple things looked familiar but I was not certain. They told me that I had remembered a good amount for having my dominant side shut down. I hadn't remembered a lot, that was for sure, but for the dominant side being essentially "off", I did remember more than they seemed to think I would, which was a pleasant surprise to me. I wondered if that would be good news? I thought to myself that the test had went well and wondered how long it would be before I would get any kind of results. They told me to just relax for a while and they would be back in a bit. So, I just stayed there, laying on the table, wondering what would come. Wondering if my last step would set me on the path to neurosurgery, wondering how long it would take for me to find out if I would become eligible to have my life changed. Hoping it wouldn't take weeks, or even months. I knew the test seemed complex, so I didn't dare hope it would be less than a week. I hoped it wouldn't be too long to hear back. I was anxious.

After a little while, they walked back in the room. "So, we looked over everything and you passed. Congratulations, you did great." I just looked at them. I couldn't believe it. There was no way that was it. It couldn't be that simple, at least I didn't think so in my mind. I said, "what do you mean?" They told me I did great. As far as the WADA test was concerned, I was a good surgical candidate. They would forward the results to my epileptologist so she could continue with the process. They said that they were confident I was good to go. I could not believe it! I was done! That was it! I asked what would happen next. They told me since that was the last step of the process to select a candidate for surgery, my epileptologist would set me up for a consultation to meet with a surgeon, to go over what he or she would want to do during the operation, what to expect, and then we would make the final decision together, as a team, the surgeon and me. If we decided together that we wanted to do it, we would set a surgery date. I couldn't believe it. I was on my way. I couldn't wait to talk to my epileptologist! Wow. It was real. I was probably going to have a chance. If the surgeon agreed, I was going to have brain surgery.

I got a call from my epileptologist. She congratulated me! She told me that she had to re-present my case to the multidisciplinary epilepsy conference, but believed everything would be good. We had great evidence at that point. There was a conference soon after. She would contact me again shortly and give me the results. I anxiously awaited the phone call. It didn't take long to hear back. When I did, it was the news I was hoping for. They thought it was time to move forward. It was time for me to go meet a surgeon. She told about the type of surgery I would be having. It was going to be a right temporal lobectomy. She told me the surgeons name and assured me he was/is awesome. She said his office would call me very soon to set up a consult. I was a little nervous, but also, honestly, excited. The day I had been waiting for had come. I had just found out I was truly a surgical candidate. She also said that during the conference, the experts, including the surgeon himself gave me in the ballpark, based on my case, about a 60-70% chance of becoming seizure free after the surgery. That was leaps and bounds above the odds of ever finding a medication that would work for me, statistically speaking, after all the failed drug trials that I had been through up until then. At that point, I was averaging one seizure a week. I would take it! Hands down. I was ready. I couldn't wait to meet the man and see what he had to say. I was hoping he was as nice and genuine as most of the people I had been meeting along the way, unlike the first neurologist I met at the beginning of my journey. I worried a little that the surgeon would be like him. I would have to wait and see. I didn't have to wait long though. I received the phone call shortly after speaking to my epileptologist. The surgeon's office called and set up an appointment. It was finally time to meet the man that would change my life forever.

Chapter 10. Surgery road.

I wasn't sure if Christina would want to hear what the surgeon had to say that day. This was all very unfamiliar territory for us. I thought that it may be a frightening experience for her to hear what he was planning to do to me. I know that I would want to hear every detail if she was going through something like that, but, we are different people, and I wanted to give her the opportunity to sit it out in case it was going to be too hard on her. I didn't know if she would want to hear about the operation itself in detail. So, I asked her, and I offered her an out. She wanted to go. So that was settled. We made the plans accordingly and waited for the date, which wasn't much of a wait at all. I was surprised. We only had to wait around a week and a half.

Finally, I felt as though the day I had been waiting for had arrived. The day I would find out if I was going to have brain surgery. Christina and I woke up in the morning and got ready. I slept well for someone that was going to find out potentially life changing news the next day. I do remember having a dream that he decided to do the surgery that day, and had performed it in a bizarre setting, a fully metal, rusty room of some sort. That was interesting, I found it quite funny. I woke up kind of wondering if I had a seizure. Sometimes I had vivid dreams like that when I had nocturnal seizures from time to time, and I had wondered if I had one that night, but I was not sure. I didn't wake up doing any of my normal seizure "activities", or feeling my post-ictal feelings, so I dismissed it as a vivid dream, caused by an overactive imagination due to the events to come that day.

After getting ready, we got in the car and headed down to his office, across the street from where the operation would be performed if we all agreed to move forward. We left with plenty of extra time in case there was traffic, or any other issue on the way. We ended up getting there early, which in my book is always good. I am always happy to sit in a waiting room for some time, collecting my thoughts, going over my notes and questions, trying to come up with any last-minute inquiries for the doctor, while thinking for a bit before something big like that. Before long though, the nurse came out and called us back early, awesome! She brought us into a room and sat us down in his office. She told us that he would be in shortly. I had my seizure diary that I keep, per my epileptologists request, and in it, I also had questions for him that we had come up with.

After the nurse left, Christina and I sat and talked for a few of minutes. We mostly discussed what we should ask the surgeon. I quietly wondered to myself if my childhood brain surgeon "stereotypes" would fit. I have always imagined them as coming off slightly eccentric, cocky, or maybe just so hyper intelligent that you would be able to sort of see their level of human intellectual superiority written all over them. I remember thinking it was a silly thought, but I was finally going to meet a

Jimmy Golden. MY GOLDEN MIND, A JOURNEY THROUGH EPILEPSY AND BRAIN SURGERY

brain surgeon for the first time. It was something I had always wanted to do, but obviously not in that context. All those things were going through my mind during those several minutes before he came in. Also, the elephant in the room. Brain surgery. I was HOPING this man would perform brain surgery on me. It seemed strange to me to want brain surgery, but I did, and I was ready for it at that point.

After a knock, and we replied with a "come in", the door opened, and in walked the man that changed the course of my life, and by doing so, influence the lives of all of those of whom I hold most dear. He walked in casually, with his white doctor's coat on. He had short brown hair, with a beard, not intimidating looking at all. My first thought was that he looked very friendly. He first walked up to me. He shook my hand, then Christina's. While doing so, he introduced himself. "Hi, ------- --------, good to meet you." He said the same to Christina as he shook her hand. I noticed right away that introduced himself by his first and last name only, rather than by his professional title followed by last name. That caught my attention. I thought it was interesting. Not that I think there is anything wrong, at all, with doctors referring to themselves as "doctor". Doctors, after all, more than deserve that, after the unbelievably hard work and dedication they put in to earn that title. I just automatically thought he was being humble.

After exchanging some pleasantries, he sat down and said "Okay, so tell me Jimmy, do you know how you ended up in my office, and why you are here today?" Now, I look at that on paper, and it may sound a little abrasive almost, but I assure you, it wasn't. He seemed to be gauging how familiar I was with my own case, and by doing so, attempting to not only avoid wasting all our time by going over a bunch of things we all already knew, but to also avoid making us feel as though we were "uninformed patients", if that makes sense. I got the impression he was trying to avoid insulting us by taking that step. He wanted to only tell us things we needed to hear, in my opinion, so that we didn't feel as though he were treating us like we hadn't been paying enough attention to things we should have been paying attention to or something. No need to go through every step and explain everything if we already knew. So, I told him. I quickly made it clear I knew what was going on.

He told me that I was right about the process leading up to me ending up in his office, and that, I was indeed in his office because I was deemed a surgical candidate.

At that point, he started getting into the things that were more surgery related. Not that there was anything wrong with what he had already said. He told us if we had any questions while he was talking, to ask. He explained the odds of seizure freedom. He talked to me about my seizures. He showed us some of my MRI scans and talked to us about them being clean, and then explained how, since they were, they used all the other evidence to build the case, and eventually became certain that they knew exactly where the spot was that my seizures were coming from. He was great, Christina and I loved him instantly. He didn't rush us at all. He answered all our questions and spent a lot of time with us. He was very caring and kind.

The main questions I had for him that day were simple, and I could lay them out for him all at once because he had explained everything so well. "Is my case cut and dry for you? Was it easy for you to make the decision to want to operate? Is there anything that makes you question doing this temporal lobectomy? If I were a family member of yours, would you want to perform this surgery?" His responses made me feel even more comfortable. He told me that the decision was clear. There had been absolutely nothing at all that didn't point to the area that they believed to be the focal point. He said every step of the process pointed to the same area of my brain being the culprit. He had no doubt that surgery was the best route for me to take, and he would absolutely recommend it to a family member. He, in fact, strives to treat all his patients no different than he would treat one of his own family members. He wouldn't do something to a patient, that he wouldn't do to someone in his own family. I was honestly almost sold on surgery before walking in the room. I was tired, I was drained, I was burned out and browbeaten a little. It was settled then and there though, after hearing those words. I asked him when we could do it. He asked when we would want to. I told him I was ready when he was. It was December. He asked if we wanted to do it before or after the holidays. We both agreed it would be better to do it after. We didn't want to burden our families with the stress of brain surgery recovery during the holiday season. He looked at his calendar. "How about January 19, 2017?" That was the next month. I told him it worked for me. It was settled. We shook hands and we got up. He walked us out and we chatted a little. He took us to his receptionist to have me booked for the operation. It was a done deal. She scheduled me for two things that day, my pre-op, and my right temporal lobectomy. It was finally determined, after all this time and testing. I was officially going to have brain surgery, I was going to have a right temporal lobectomy on January the 19th, 2017. I had just met the man that was going to change the course of my life forever. I just hoped that it would work.

Before heading to the appointment, I, of course, had told my parents that I was heading down. They knew it was that day, and they had high hopes for me. They wanted what was best for me. I had told my friends too. Everyone wanted to know the outcome. I honestly didn't expect that I would get a date that day. My Mom, on the other hand, told me I likely would. She was right, as usual. I kind of thought, even if I did get a date, it would be at least months down the road before I could get in.

Jimmy Golden. MY GOLDEN MIND, A JOURNEY THROUGH EPILEPSY AND BRAIN SURGERY

Some of the tests, like the WADA and the MEG took a reasonable amount of time to get scheduled, so in my mind, it was only reasonable to expect a long delay to have neurosurgery. I called my Mom on the way home and told her the news. She was happy for me. She knew that is what I wanted, and it was the best chance at having a seizure free life. I couldn't help but feel like she seemed a little off though, like maybe she seemed slightly emotional. I never asked her about it. Maybe I will someday. Maybe the news that your son is going to have brain surgery is a large pill to swallow. It could be that she was just happy for me too. I'm not sure. I may have been imagining it. I let my friends know. I told Aldo, he was excited. I let my friend Ron know, the race car one, he couldn't have been happier, I even text messaged Nick. We told Christina's parents. This was huge. I couldn't wait. I know that may sound strange. Not being able to wait for brain surgery. I was excited though. Every step of the way, other than my first neurologist, had been great. I was sure that the operation would be as good as brain surgery could possibly be. Again, trying to see the glass as half full.

Jimmy Golden. MY GOLDEN MIND, A JOURNEY THROUGH EPILEPSY AND BRAIN SURGERY

Christina was graduated by then, but she was still working full time, so it was going to be difficult for her to take care of me. We had considered just going and getting married at the courthouse at that point. We were already engaged, we had been together forever. We thought, "Maybe we should just make it official, FMLA after surgery would be a big help." I kind of made the decision. I was the one with epilepsy. I did not want to take away the wedding that I wanted her to be able to have. The wedding that I felt like she deserved to have, because I had fallen ill. I didn't want to get married at the courthouse just so she could take care of me. I wasn't going to do it. I decided we would wait until we could plan it the way we were originally planning, and I did my best to smoothly talk her into agreeing with me, without her realizing that was why. She will soon enough, after she reads my book, obviously. The way I saw it, we had waited this long already. We would wait until the time is right, like we have for so long before.

My parents are awesome, they had recently retired and moved to Oregon, but kindly, my Mom volunteered to come down a week before my pre-op and stay at our house. They said she would stay through the surgery, then for as long as we needed her to help take care of me, and until everything was squared away. Awesome. What a relief! Plus, to put the icing on the cake, Christina is so busy with being a speech and language pathologist, that she doesn't cook much. She is just always on the move, she frequently must take work home, and if she isn't working, she goes to the gym. I was usually the cook before all this started. So, when my Mom said she was coming, I was thinking to myself, "dinner! Yay mom! Score!"

While waiting for my pre-op, I tried to keep busy. I was a little anxious, but not as bad as one might think. My friend Ron called me up one day and asked me if I wanted to go with him to his lake house, not long before my pre-op, shortly before my parents were scheduled to arrive, to hang out with him while he worked on some trim on his boat dock. At that point in my life, I was always happy to get out of the house! I told him I would love to go!

As I previously mentioned, Ron had made a bit of a habit of this. He knew I was at home and alone during the week, pretty much all the time, so anytime he was going to be off, and was going to be doing something, he would try and invite me to get me out of the house. I really appreciated that. More than he probably realizes. He picked me up early in the morning, and we headed out to his lake house. It is a little over an hour or so from where we both live. We usually talk race cars, work, friends and politics. We always have a good time. We were there for a few hours and he was working on re painting his boat dock trim. I helped him where I could, mostly handing him things, holding things for him, stuff like that. I couldn't do much. The seizures put me at too much of a risk. Especially around water. I mostly sat there and talked with him.

My phone rang. I recognized the area code. It was where the hospital is located. I answered it. It was indeed the hospital, and they needed to do one last test before surgery to help with the procedure. They needed one more CAT scan. They wanted me to come down as soon as possible. They asked if I could come right then. I, of course, couldn't drive. I didn't know what to do. We were a good two and a half hours away from the hospital, without traffic. I hated even the thought of asking Ron to take me down there. To pull him away from his work. I already always felt like a burden on everyone, but this was way worse than usual. He asked what it was, and I told him. He asked when they wanted to do it, and I told him they wanted to do it right then. I felt terrible, I didn't know what to think. He said, "No problem, lets clean this up and we will head down right away, tell her we will be down there as soon as possible." I asked him if he was sure. He told me "absolutely Junior, no problem, none of this stuff means anything, we can finish it any time." That is who Ron is. He would do anything for anybody at the drop of a hat, no questions asked. Ron has taken me all over the place. Between other types of doctor visits, post ops, races, building my race car, you name it, Ron has treated me like a son, and I hope one day I can repay him somehow. I wonder, also, if you noticed that he called me "Junior". Ron is where calling one another "junior" came from. There are quite a few of us now, friends and colleges from the same place, who call one another that, and it all came from Ron. I like to think it will go on for long after he retires. A sort of legacy in a way.

So just like that, we packed up all his stuff, jumped in his car and headed all the way down to the hospital. A good two and a half hours away, for a CAT scan that may have taken all of twenty minutes. I was thankful he was there to help me out that day, but I felt terrible I had to have him take me like that. He knows I would do the same for him at a moment's notice, but that didn't make me feel any better. There are times where you just can't help but feel bad for having to have people run you around all the time. No matter how much they assure you they are there for you. I sure have been lucky to have been surrounded by such good people throughout my journey.

My Mom arrived on January 9, 2017. One day before my pre-op. Ten days and counting before my surgery. Crazy! I had been off work so long already that it felt like I didn't even have a job anymore, although, they were holding my position for me, luckily. It was good to see my Mom. She flew down and got a rental car to drive to our house. We would have picked her up from the airport, but because Christina was working and we are good drive from Los Angeles, my Mom insisted on driving herself up. She turned the rental back in by our house, and would use my truck while staying in our extra bedroom for the extent of her stay, however long it ended up being. My Mom didn't want Christina to have to drive to LA on a work night to go get her.

It was finally the day of the pre-op. I was ready. My Mom drove me down, Christina had to work that day. My pre-op was in the morning, early. It was on January 10, 2017. It was not really going to be a big deal. We met with the anesthesiologist to go over the process and make sure we didn't have any questions or medication concerns. We went over what I needed to do prior to the surgery. We also met with the surgeon so that he could meet my Mom, since she would be taking care of me after surgery. He explained what to expect and went over everything with both of us. He wanted us to be well informed about what would happen after the surgery.

The pre-op went very well. My Mom and I both liked the anesthesiologist. I do not do well with opioid pain medications, they make me very nauseous. So, she talked to us about that, and told us that she would do everything she could to prevent nausea. My Mom also agreed with how Christina and I felt about my surgeon. She agreed that he was very kind and caring and that I was in extraordinarily good hands. He treated her the same way he treated us. I also had to go and sign all the paperwork for the hospital stay, and for the surgery itself that day. All the typical stuff you would sign before any surgery. I have had several knee surgeries, so I was used to it. I knew what to expect. They told me to head over to the laboratory afterward, to have my blood work done. Even that was a pleasant experience. The phlebotomist hit it right on the mark, no problem. Great day! I was officially on my way. Only thing left was the surgery itself! No more testing, no more anything. Just go home, wait for Christina to arrive, hang out with my mom and wait ten days for the operation! Hopefully, I wouldn't have too many seizures in the meantime. To think, after those ten days, there was a possibility I would never have another seizure!

My Mom and I left the hospital feeling good. That was it. I was waiting for my surgery. We were talking while she was driving. I don't really remember what we were talking about, but I do remember, as she was getting on the freeway to head back home, my phone rang. I looked at the caller ID, and it was

Jimmy Golden. MY GOLDEN MIND, A JOURNEY THROUGH EPILEPSY AND BRAIN SURGERY

Christina. I thought, "oh that's nice, she is calling to see how the pre-op went." Boy, was I wrong.

I answered the phone. "Hello?" She said, "I was in a car accident, I am at ----- ------- hospital. I think I'm okay, but I'm sore, and I was knocked out. They are going to do tests on me. I have a collar on, and my car was upside down and I couldn't get out." No way. I couldn't believe it. She had been in a terrible car accident on her way to work. Long story short, it had been raining, something happened, and her small four door vehicle veered off the road, off an embankment, nosedived, did a front flip, and landed upside down. She ended up trapped in her vehicle, stuck hanging upside down, and was knocked unconscious upon impact. Luckily, a fellow good Samaritan had witnessed the accident and stopped. There was no cell phone service in that area because of the mountains, so he helped her. Another good Samaritan drove to the nearby ranger station to get help. They came and called for an ambulance. They deemed her as having head trauma, and sent her to the closest trauma center. She ended up having a concussion. Honestly, looking at the location, the lack of cell phone service, the lack of usual traffic that time of day, the fact that her car was difficult to spot from the road do to where it landed, the horrific damage to her totaled vehicle, I would say she is honestly lucky to have survived that accident. Even more than that, to have walked away with only the injuries she did. Still, we were all terribly worried about her. I was not familiar with the trauma center she was taken to by the ambulance, so I had to look it up on my phone. My Mom drove us there right away.

I never mentioned this to anyone, but things like that are what really makes this condition difficult on us, especially those of us who are adults. I hid my feelings from my Mother that day in the car, but I was, one more time, engulfed by the dark shadow of epilepsy. The happiness I was feeling about getting ready for surgery was crushed by the feelings of uselessness that came following that phone call. I fight feelings like those, but they would always come back. You or the person battling epilepsy in your life will go through the same cycles. The problem was, I had thoughts racing through my mind telling me, "Here you are, and the woman you care about more than anyone else in the world is lying in a hospital bed, and you are riding in the passenger seat, basically useless, unable to do anything, relying on somebody else. What would have happened if someone wouldn't have been here to help?" Without being able to drive that day, I felt as if my Mother hadn't been there, I would have failed Christina that day, because of my disorder, and it hurt me. It darkened my overall being just a little bit more. From the beginning of this journey, I have always felt that I was constantly fighting a war with myself to not go "permanently dark" inside. Every time something like that really hit home with me, I lost a little bit of my "light" if you will, or what makes me a happy person. I fought that battle every day. I hid it from most of the world, I didn't see any reason to burden anyone with my struggles. My battle with the part of epilepsy everyone can see, and must deal with, was enough of a burden for everyone else already, as far as I was concerned.

We got to the hospital as soon as we could. It was on our way home, but still out of the way, so to speak, so we could get there quickly. While on our way there, I contacted her mother at work, and I informed her of the accident. She immediately left, and headed to the hospital. We were also able to get a message to her father Ray, who was also at work, and came. What a crazy start to 2017. She was eventually released that evening with instructions to follow up with her primary care physician. I couldn't help but feel as if we really dodged a bullet. To walk away from such a horrific accident like that was a wonderful thing. I know I am wearing this out a little, but again, the glass was half full.

Fairly soon after, Christina was starting to feel better, although the effects of her concussion were definitely evident. She was having some memory and concentration issues, among other things. She felt as though it made her able to relate to what I had been going through a little more, because, of course, I had been having lots of the same problems she was now experiencing, for a long time. I felt bad for her. I knew she wasn't feeling well. I knew what she was going through, in a sense. Her doctor made her take a little time off work because she wanted her to get lots of rest and relaxation. Her job requires a lot of concentration and thought processing, and the doctor didn't want her doing much of that while her brain healed from the concussion. So, we spent a little time with my Mom, relaxing, recovering, enjoying some home cooked meals, and preparing for surgery.

I woke up one morning, and after brushing my teeth and getting dressed, I went to go see if my mom had woken up. I walked out of the master bedroom, and my Mom was standing in the hallway outside of the bathroom. I told her good morning. I thought it was odd that she was up so early. She quickly told me "I invited my boyfriend over, I hope you don't mind". I laughed. I obviously knew she was joking. My parents have been married for over thirty years. My Dad was up in Oregon. She pointed in the bedroom, so I looked in there, and there was my Dad, sitting on the bed. He had come down to stay with us too. What a nice surprise. I hadn't seen him in a while! So now I got to spend time with both of my parents during all of this. I had thought that my Dad would just come down for the surgery only. He ended up staying the entire time my Mom did, which was great.

A little less than one week before surgery, all four of us had just finished eating a late breakfast. Christina, my parents and myself. Christina and I were in the kitchen, and my parents were in the living room talking and sitting on the couch. The doorbell rang. My Dad asked if I wanted him to get it, but I told him I would. In the area where we live, we get a lot of people trying to sell things door to door. I am used to it. I don't mind, everyone must make a living after all. I always answer the door for Christina just in case it is someone of concern. I looked out the peep hole and nobody was there. I opened the door and looked, and there was a large cardboard document envelope on the ground. I figured it was either from the hospital, from my work, or had something to do with Christina's work. I read the Label on it, and my chest immediately felt heavy, I knew what it was, at least somewhat. I walked back in the house, and like I had grown used to doing, I hid my emotions. I don't remember who, but someone asked what it was, and I came up with some excuse. I told them it was from work or something like that. I don't really remember now. I said I had to go to the bathroom, and I went to the master bedroom. The package label really said, "WH-OFFICE OF RECORDS MGT", and it was from Washington DC. I knew it then and there. I didn't know what kind, but I had received a response to the letter I had sent to president Barack Obama some time back before my WADA test.

I walked in the master bedroom. I closed and locked the door, and I sat on the bed. I looked at the packaging material for a moment and reread it all. I was shocked that I had received anything at all. I wondered to myself what could possibly be inside. I asked myself "could this be something else? Is there any other reason I would receive something from Washington DC, from something that appears to be from the White House, and shipped next day air?" I was having a hard time coming up with a good excuse. The package was labeled "Extremely Urgent" in red letters. I started thinking about the material I had read online about who might respond to citizens for the president. Sometimes people will receive a bit of a "thank you for writing the president" card type of thing. That is what I have read anyway. Sometimes people receive letters from someone in his staff, even signed by them and all. There are even a very rare lucky few, whom receive a letter back from the president himself, hand signed in ink! I was just happy to have received anything though. I told myself no matter what was in there, I was going to be happy that I received a reply! I caught myself imagining opening it, and finding a letter from the president himself. I shook that fantasy off. That would be like winning the lottery. I was crazy to even think that. I needed to get it over with. I started worrying that my family would think that I had been gone too long, and would think I had a seizure.

I carefully tore the cardboard strip back to open the package. Inside was another package. It had my name and address on it. It was a sealed document sized envelope and it said, "first class do not bend". I carefully opened it. Inside was a thick piece of stiff cardboard, with a letter on it. It is printed on an off white, thicker than usual, high quality, almost resume style piece of paper. It is a little smaller than a piece of computer paper, but not tiny. On the top of the page, it has an eagle seal imprinted on it, and below the seal it says, "THE WHITE HOUSE" and "WASHINGTON" printed in royal blue. I read the first line of the letter and got the chills. Not only was this not a thank you card, but yes, this was an actual letter. I wish I could publish the letter, but I would need permission to do that. It was him. It was Barack Obama. My letter had made it all the way to the president's desk. In the letter, he informed me he had read my letter personally. He thanked me for sharing my story with him. He told me how letters like mine have helped to keep him up to date throughout his time as president of the United States. He also told me that he and Michelle would keep myself and my Fiancée in their thoughts, and wished us the best in our difficult time, among several other things of course. It was an actual, real, full-fledged personal letter. Also, at the bottom, it is hand signed, in ink. I couldn't believe it. I was holding a letter, written personally to me, from the president of the United States. The glass wasn't half full that day, it was over flowing, all over the floor, flooding the house!

I walked out into the kitchen, where Christina had been cleaning, while holding the letter. I had slid it back into the envelope. I had her come over to the kitchen table with me. I told her I wanted to show her something. I had her make sure her hands were dry and clean. I remember her seeming to think it was an odd request. Remember, up to that point, I had never told a single person in the world I had written my letter to the president, including Christina. I had only mentioned, quite some time before I wrote it, that one day, I would like to write one to him, and left it at that. I took it out of the envelope and I showed it to her. She read through it, and it took her a second to take it in. Since I had never told her I wrote to him, it seemed to be somewhat confusing for a second. When it dawned on her what it was, when she recognized the signature, when she recognized his speech patterns ("folks like you"), when she realized he said, "it has been a privilege to serve as your president", she couldn't believe it. She was so happy for me. It couldn't have come at a better time for me honestly. It gave me some extra encouragement. No, honestly, it gave me a lot of extra encouragement going into brain surgery. There is something about the president of the United States personally wishing you the best, telling you that you are in his, and his wife's thoughts during your difficult time, about one week prior to life changing brain surgery, that just makes you feel better about everything you are going through. I really do wish I could thank him personally for sending me that letter, because it really did make a big difference in my life. It uplifted my battered, weathered and browbeaten overall being at that point, with everything Christina and I had been going through. That letter was truly a precious gift, given at a perfect moment. It put some spring back in my step, it put some light back into my life that had been slowly, partially extinguished by epilepsy, and I really needed that before surgery. That letter is now my prized possession in life. I truly mean that. Other than people, I care about nothing that exists physically in my life more.

After showing Christina, I brought it into the living room where my parents were sitting and talking. I had asked Christina to not say anything too loud, because my parents did not know yet. I told my parents I had something to show them. I, just like with Christina, made sure their hands were clean. They read the letter and, naturally, thought it was awesome. Next, of course, everyone was curious about the letter that I had sent to him. I told them that I had not told anyone about it because I had always imagined that I would not be lucky enough to get a response. I knew how long the odds were. I had done the research. I still couldn't believe it. I told them I would be happy to let them read it, so one by one, they all did. Afterward, my Dad drove me to an arts and crafts store to pick out a nice frame.

Jimmy Golden. MY GOLDEN MIND, A JOURNEY THROUGH EPILEPSY AND BRAIN SURGERY

I wanted to frame it right away so that nothing would happen to it. I wanted to get it protected. What a day. To think, I almost didn't write that letter. I was too worried about failure. I didn't want to feel like I was rejected because I knew how the odds were stacked against me. I took a chance though. Just like with writing this book. You should too. No matter who you are. If you want to do something in life, go for it. Don't sit around and make excuses about why it won't work out for you. I almost gave in to those excuses, but I decided not to. Now, I have a letter hanging on my wall from the president that I will cherish forever, and it gives me inspiration every single day. It especially helps me on my bad days. It is all because I decided not to let the darkness extinguish my light completely, and I went for it. I put myself out there and I took a shot. My next gamble was to come in less than one week. The odds were in my favor that time, and what I could walk away with could change the course of my life forever. I really wanted the win, and I had been fighting to get into the game for about a year, and it was coming up on game day. Thanks to my support group made up of family, friends, coworkers, doctors, and now, in my mind, the president of the

United States of America, I was readier than I had ever been. I was feeling as good as anyone could feel before brain surgery. I was ready. Bring it on. I'm not scared of some surgery!

Jimmy Golden. MY GOLDEN MIND, A JOURNEY THROUGH EPILEPSY AND BRAIN SURGERY

Jimmy Golden. MY GOLDEN MIND, A JOURNEY THROUGH EPILEPSY AND BRAIN SURGERY

Chapter 11. Surgery

January 18, 2017. That was the day it officially started, at least in my mind. Since I had to check in at the hospital for my operation at 6:30 in the morning, and it was in Los Angeles, which is a little over an hour from us, we decided to get a couple of hotel rooms that were walking distance from the hospital. We didn't want to end up being late because of L.A. traffic or an accident of some kind on the freeway in the morning. Christina and I had got one room just for the night prior to the surgery, and my parents were going to get a room for the approximate duration of my stay in the hospital, so that they had a place to stay down there, and anyone could go there if need be, including

Christina. Christina was back at work by then, so she was, other than the day of my surgery, going to be traveling back and forth to come and visit with me. I didn't want her to be down there with me the whole time. I felt it was unnecessary. I was told I would be very sleepy and would not be doing much but sleeping after the operation and, for a couple of days, would be in the intensive care unit, so visiting would be limited anyway. The ICU stay is a precautionary measure to prevent infection and to make sure you are well monitored from my understanding.

The night before the surgery, we checked into our hotel rooms and wanted to get some dinner. I had to eat my last meal, and drink my last liquid by a certain time. So, we wanted to make sure we had plenty of time to do that, which we did. I wanted to eat something mild, because I didn't want to risk having any acid reflux problems during my operation. I sometimes get heartburn. There was a Subway right around the corner, so I thought we should just walk over and eat that. That was nice and mild for me. I got my usual ham and turkey on flat bread with avocado, and nothing else at all. Christina thinks I am weird, but that is what I like on sandwiches. I have simple taste.

Jimmy Golden. MY GOLDEN MIND, A JOURNEY THROUGH EPILEPSY AND BRAIN SURGERY

Many of the people at the sandwich shops in town often remember me when we go buy sandwiches, and I tell her it's because I am nice and talkative, and she tells me it's because I order weird sandwiches. We laugh about this all the time. Maybe one day I will ask them, and we will see who is right.

We all headed back to the hotel rooms. I told my parents they could eat with us, but they didn't. They told us to eat and then go to sleep. I feel like the real reason was a combination of two things. I believe my Mom was starting to get a little worried about the operation, and it would have been hard for her to sit down and eat with us. It would have been a little too much of a "last meal" kind of setting, and also, I think they knew Christina was worried and anxious and wanted to give us alone time. That was a kind gesture from them, but it was not necessary. We would have been happy to spend time with them of course.

Christina did well that night. Better than I thought she would honestly. She only just before we fell asleep, had a bit of an emotional episode. Christina is an intelligent, educated professional. She has a master's degree in a field that often deals with people whom have the same condition that I have. She understands it, and I think that helps. It was still hard on her though, and brain surgery is a tough pill to swallow for anyone who loves somebody. She understood the statistics. She knew that the chances of something going wrong were so low that they were nearly negligible. That didn't matter to her though when she looked into my eyes the night before brain surgery, and I understood that. I could only imagine being in her situation. The uncertainty that she had lived through with me at the beginning, then the terrible tonic clonic she witnessed, the diagnosis, me losing my driver's license and not being able to work, all the other complex partials she had witnessed, then all the testing, and at that point, knowing she was going to watch me be carted off the next day to have part of my brain removed. It must all have been hard on her. I understood her fear. With tears in her eyes, she told me "I am afraid to lose you." I felt for her that night in the hotel room. I did my best to comfort her. I told her "I am not going anywhere my love, I have too much left to do. I have too much left to accomplish in life. We still must get married. Like it or not, you are stuck with me, I am right here, and I will be just fine. I am not afraid, and you shouldn't be either. It's going to be okay, trust me, I can feel it. I'm not done yet." I held on to her, and we drifted off to sleep. My final night with a full brain.

My alarm went off. It woke me up. I slept well. I had anticipated having a hard time sleeping, but I didn't. Honestly, I had been treated so well, I trusted everyone so much, I trusted the surgeon so much, I was at ease. I felt comfortable. I got up and got ready, and so did Christina. After we were ready, we met with my parents. We headed to the hospital. My Mom drove us. We were in my truck. We could have walked there, but it was raining some, and it made more sense to drive. I had a bag with my medications and everything for my stay. It was still dark out. I could tell my Mom was nervous and uneasy. I felt sorry for her. I could tell by the way she was driving. She was doing her best to hide it, but she wasn't doing well with all that was happening, emotionally. I think it was a little difficult for my Dad too, he is just less emotional than my Mom. He hides things better than she does. He is more like me that way. When things come out though, they can really come out, again, just like me.

We got to the hospital, they got their visitors passes and I checked in. Now all there was to do was to wait to be called. We were a little early. They came out on schedule and called me back. I gave everyone a hug, and went on back. They said they would be able to go back there in a bit, after I was set up and in the holding area before surgery. I felt good. I really didn't feel nervous. I was feeling good to go. My biggest concern through all of this was still that the surgery wouldn't work.

After they got me in the back room, some very friendly nurses came in and introduced themselves. They told me to change into a hospital gown and socks. They gave me the privacy to do so. They gave me a bag for my belongings. After, they set me up with some IV catheters in the top of my hands. They did a great job. No pain, and they hit them right on the mark.

Once I was in bed and set up, they let my family come in. I ended up meeting several people. I met a second neurosurgeon who would be assisting in the surgery. He was very nice as well. We talked to the anesthesiologist again, and

Jimmy Golden. MY GOLDEN MIND, A JOURNEY THROUGH EPILEPSY AND BRAIN SURGERY

basically everyone who would take part in the surgery. Just like with all surgeries, they confirmed why I was there, which side the surgery was going to be on. They marked the side of my head with a pen. They asked me a little about my seizures. I had lots of interesting things to talk about with people. My surgeon himself, however, was preforming another operation at the time, so I didn't see him at first, and I saw him a little later. My surgery ended up starting just a little bit behind schedule because of the previous surgery he had performed. Both the surgeon himself, and many other of the medical professionals apologized numerous times for the short delay. I had no problem with it at all. This man was changing and or saving lives. The way I saw it, I didn't care how long it took him. I wanted what was best for everyone, including the person whom he was helping before me. I just hoped he or she had a successful surgery. I remember sitting in the waiting room, people asking how I felt. I honestly felt just fine. Of course, I was slightly nervous, but nowhere near what you would think someone might feel prior to brain surgery. I was honestly a little board at times. The medical personnel seemed to notice my calm demeanor. Several of them mentioned it. They did it in a complementary and tactful way, careful not to trigger fear or anything, not that I think they could have. I knew exactly what I was getting into already. I just trusted the hospital, and the people in it. Everyone since the first neurologist had been so amazing, I just knew this was the right choice, and I was in incredible hands. I didn't feel I had any reason to be worried. It was honestly all mildly interesting to me at that point. Kind of weird, yeah, I know. Honestly though, it really isn't as scary as one might imagine.

So, Before I knew it, it was time. The moment I had been longing for, the moment I had hoped would eventually come, had become reality. They rolled me out into the hall. They let my family walk with me to a point. Then, it was time to say, "good luck, and I will see you soon!" So, we did. I told them I loved them, and I would see them in a few hours! I waved at them and they rolled me into the operating room.

I was immediately impressed by two things. Temperature, and what I was seeing. It was cold in there. I honestly thought it felt good though. They rolled my cart over next to another one. They told me I was going to be put onto that one. So, several people helped and, after a count, I was moved to the other table. They gave me some medication. I could feel it starting shortly after. I have had several knee surgeries before, so I knew what to expect during the process. They told me what it was before hand, but I don't recall now. It calms you down and makes you feel like you have had some alcohol. I was calm anyway, but it feels nice, I didn't mind. I told the woman that it felt great in there. She responded "I think you are the only person who has ever told me that. Usually people tell me they are freezing!" She thought it was funny. It was quite cold of course. Operating rooms are cold. She was very friendly. She told me they were going to give me some blankets anyway, if I didn't mind, to keep me from shivering. I didn't mind of course. I told her the room looked extraordinarily expensive. She laughed again. She told me it was. It was full of monitors and crazy looking equipment and scanners. It reminded me of the inside of a space ship. I thought it was cool. No pun intended.

After a little more prepping, my surgeon came in. He talked to me for a couple of minutes. He promised he was going to take good care of me. I told him I knew he would, and I appreciated what he was doing for me. He said he would see me soon, and he went to get ready. They moved me over to the other side of the room. I knew the time was near. Since I had been through several surgeries before, I was familiar enough with the routine to sense it. I was prepped and ready. I knew they would do a few more things like prep my head for the doctor, put my skull in a device that locates it in an exact location, and insert a urine catheter, but they would do those things after I was put under anesthesia. The nice woman who had been laughing at me, came over with a mask. She told me "This is just oxygen, I want you to breath some for a minute. Please breathe deeply for me when I put the mask on okay?" She put the mask over my mouth and nose. I told her, "this isn't my first rodeo, I know what you're doing to me". I smiled at her. She tried not to smile as I looked up at her. She was caught, she knew it. I started taking deep breaths. My last conscious breaths with a full brain. That is the last thing I remember before surgery.

I don't remember my exact first memory after the surgery. I just remember little bits and fragments of things. I was medicated and extremely tired. My first memories are very hazy. I know that my friend Aldo, Ron and his wife Kelly, Christina's parents, my friend Garrett, and of course everyone that was already there all visited. That was very nice of all of them to make the trip. I wished I could have engaged with them more, but I was certainly out of it at that point. I don't even remember how I felt honestly, I just know they were there, and I was exhausted. I wish I could say otherwise, but at that point after the surgery, I don't remember a word that was said. That isn't because anything was wrong, it is just because you are still so out of it from the anesthesia and medications you are on, and your brain is trying to recover. It is completely normal to feel that way. They told us I would feel that way before, and had and told everyone not to worry about how I acted after the surgery. They said I would basically be unresponsive for a while. I was.

As time progressed, I started feeling more and more cognizant. I started feeling much more like myself. I did have a headache, but honestly, it was nowhere near what I imagined it would be. It did hurt of course, but it wasn't even as bad as a bad migraine. The pain medications they gave were sufficient at controlling the pain. I really didn't feel that pain was an issue with this surgery at all. During the consultation for the surgery, the surgeon had told me that people often tell him that arthroscopic surgeries such as ACL reconstructions in the knee are much more painful. Well, I, in fact have had an ACL reconstruction surgery, and I can tell you without a doubt that the pain from the knee surgery is much worse than the brain surgery. I ended up reporting that back to him, so he can add that to his record. One more person to add to his reporting database. Most of the pain came from the jaw area. They must cut through the muscle that controls jaw movement, so that is a little uncomfortable naturally. It makes it a little difficult to eat and speak at first, but it really isn't all that bad. Again, the medication manages the pain just fine. If I was forced to allow them to go in again, the pain, in no way would even be a factor in my decision.

    The surgery itself lasted about six and a half hours. To me, of course, it seemed to only last a split second. I felt as though I had smiled at the nice woman in the operating room who was trying not scare me with the anesthesia, I took some

Jimmy Golden. MY GOLDEN MIND, A JOURNEY THROUGH EPILEPSY AND BRAIN SURGERY

deep breaths, and then, I was instantly in recovery. The worst part of the recovery in the hospital, honestly, was nausea. As I previously mentioned, my body does not react well to opioid medications. So, the entire time I was taking them for pain, I was mildly nauseous. It wasn't terrible, but it was the most uncomfortable part for me. They did provide me with anti-nausea medication, and it worked quite well. I felt much better than I did after my Knee operations. I thought to myself, if being nauseas is the worst part of having brain surgery, I am way cool with that! I was having a bit of a difficult time eating after the surgery. I was extremely tired though, and mainly just wanted to sleep, which again, was to be expected. They had me on a soft food and liquid diet at first. I didn't mind at all. Especially since I didn't have much of an appetite anyway. I just wanted to take it easy.

I remember the first time I saw my surgeon after I became cognizant. He asked me "do you forgive me yet?" and proceeded to tell me "It won't be long before you don't want to punch me in the face". I thought it was funny, first and foremost, but naturally, I couldn't really laugh. I really appreciated that, it kind of lightened the post brain surgery mood. I was, of course, having a hard time speaking and was tired. I know I tried to respond, but can't recall how successful I was at the time. I do, however know what response went through my brain when he asked me that. The thing is, even then, in the fog and discomfort of post brain surgery confusion, the response popped into my head instantly. I know for a fact I didn't get all of what I wanted to say out that day, but, this is what I thought, and, at least, a little bit of my response is buried in here somewhere. "I am absolutely beyond grateful for this experience. The pain, and whether I stay seizure free or not are beside the point. The fact that you gave me the chance at a better life is nearly overwhelming to me, thank you, from the bottom of my heart. Also, I couldn't get myself to punch you in the face, after what you did for me, for 100,000.00$, even if you told me to." I did, in fact, make sure he got to hear that response, my full response, later in my journey. After everything he did, I found it important that he knew my answer to that question.

I was quickly feeling better and better in the hospital. It wasn't long before they downgraded me and put me in a non-

Jimmy Golden. MY GOLDEN MIND, A JOURNEY THROUGH EPILEPSY AND BRAIN SURGERY

ICU area. Everyone there treated me like gold. I was blown away how wonderful and caring everyone was. There was not a single person there whom I didn't enjoy the company or presence of. From my surgeon to the nursing staff, the therapists to the people changing the trash bins for us, and the people bringing me food. Everyone was great. As strange as it may sound, it truly wasn't really that bad of an experience. Sure, I wasn't all that comfortable, I had a headache, my jaw was uncomfortable, I was very tired, I had a hard time talking at first, I was constipated from the anesthesia, being nauseous is never fun, but I honestly expected it to be much worse. I just had brain surgery after all. They took part of my skull off and removed a section of my brain that the surgeon explained to me as being the size of four casino dice, lined up in a row, from the inside of my right temporal lobe. So, deep in my brain. I imagined I would be absolutely in terrible pain and completely miserable. I really wasn't. I had felt better, sure, but I would choose to feel that way over knee surgery. I would probably choose to feel that way over a bad flu with a bad headache honestly. I was happy with the way I was feeling. After what I had just been through, I felt lucky. It may have taken a little while, a day or maybe two, to really start coming around and communicating well, but that was just fine with me. I was just too tired at first to think straight. Which again, was normal.

They checked on me constantly while I was in the hospital. Well not constantly, but you get the idea. My surgeon even made the walk from his office across the street, to the hospital, and up to the area where I was to talk to me and check on me numerous times. I really appreciated that. That is who my surgeon is though. He really is a great man. He wasn't lying when he told me in the consultation that he treated patients like an extension of his own family. My appreciation for him only continued to grow following surgery. I continued to feel better and better. They told me that because the surgeon had essentially given me a traumatic brain injury during the surgery by removing a section of brain, I was at risk of having a seizure. So, because of that, I was, for lack of better words, given a free pass on having seizures at first. If I was to have seizures directly after surgery, they would be deemed to have been caused by the surgery itself, and from the "trauma" inflicted to the brain by removing the brain matter. That meant, we didn't need to worry that the surgery was not successful if I were to have one or more of any type of seizures shortly after surgery. I didn't though. For the days following the surgery, I stayed seizure free in the hospital, feeling better and better. Soon, on the afternoon of January the 23rd, 2017, it was time. I was deemed safe and good to go. I was discharged from the hospital. It was time to go home to recover from my temporal lobectomy. It was time to start my post-surgery life.

Jimmy Golden. MY GOLDEN MIND, A JOURNEY THROUGH EPILEPSY AND BRAIN SURGERY

Chapter 12. Recovery.

"Man, she would have made a good nurse." I remember thinking that on numerous occasions about my Mom. I was incredibly lucky that she had come to help us out. She did a lot for me. She made sure I took my medications, she made sure I ate, she made sure I had ice packs, she cooked for everyone in general, she cleaned stuff. She took care of lots of things. She was a major help. Christina was working, so it really made things easier. With her being so early in her career, we really didn't want her to have to take a bunch of time off like that. My

Dad helped a lot too. He did a lot of store runs for us, he made sure I had fresh ice packs constantly (they really made me feel better during the recovery), he kept my friends up to date, he ran around the house to get things for me, and just did random things for me whenever I needed anything. I don't know what I would have done without them. I was still very tired after getting home. I wanted to sleep a lot. I spent a lot of time resting. That was basically what they told me to do. They said "if you are sleepy, sleep. Don't fight it. Sleep as much as your brain wants you to sleep." So, I did. My parents kept a good eye on me. I had lots of visitors, which was awesome. All kinds of friends, and my sisters. I had a lot of support.

Time continued to pass, slowly but surely. No seizures. I was having headaches, but they were not too bad. I was taking pain medication to keep them in check. It was the medication that they prescribed, but honestly, they were not as bad as I anticipated at all. I only took about one fourth of the pain medication as I was allotted. I am not a big fan of opioid pain medication, and I didn't really feel like I needed it too often because the pain was only bad enough for it occasionally. Mostly at night when I was laying down for long periods flat. The ice, and the small doses of medication were more than sufficient for the level of pain. The nausea had gone away because of an anti-nausea medication they had prescribed. If I took it with the pain medication, I felt just fine. I ate pretty much all soft food. Solid at that point, but soft. He had told me I could eat whatever I wanted by the time I left the hospital, but just to be careful because the more I worked my jaw, the more painful it would become, and the bigger headache I would end up with.

That was really about all there was to the recovery. My parents hung around and made sure I had everything I needed. Christina went to work, and came home when she got off. My Mom cooked us good food, and we watched some TV together. I slept a lot. I had an occupational and a physical therapist come by, sent by the insurance company, and they both told me right away they couldn't believe how well I was doing. The occupational therapist signed me off on day one because I could shower, get dressed and basically take care of myself without help, and was able to prove it to him. He was very cool. I could have survived without help honestly, but I would have been miserable, and it wouldn't have been safe. They just wanted to be sure I didn't need assistance with movement and dressing and things of that nature. The physical therapist came once a week for a while to do some exercises. She made sure I could function properly and taught me how to keep up muscle strength while recovering. She also always checked my vitals to be sure I was doing okay. She was sweet. I really enjoyed her visits. It didn't take long before she signed me off. Just like that, my therapy was over. I remember thinking, "wow, that was easy." I really was strong though. I didn't lose much of my original strength I should say. I didn't feel like I had lost anything. I was honestly stronger after surgery than I am now because of all the down time I spent sitting around between then and now. I was feeling good. I was feeling positive. I had done it. I had surgery, and after a couple weeks, I was still without a single seizure, and I hadn't even felt any depersonalization. Honestly, it was almost weird, but in a good way of course.

Before too long, I went down to see the physician's assistant for my first follow up. She was a very nice woman. She told me I looked great for someone who had just recently had the surgery I had. She, of course asked about seizures and I gladly reported I hadn't had any. At that point, that was the longest I had gone in a long time. She had to refill a couple of prescriptions for me, and she set up another appointment for me to go back down soon to have my staples removed. I was looking forward to that. I would be able to wash my head thoroughly, and shave it again. I shave my head because, well, genetics. As the old saying goes, I didn't choose this haircut, it chose me.

We continued living, all four of us together. I knew my parents wouldn't stay around for too long. I was glad they were there, but it was only a matter of time before they would have to go back to their own lives. Christina and I didn't want them to leave. They were a massive help for both of us with everything going on. I was still very tired and sleeping a lot. My Mom was still basically taking care of me. I could have been taking care of myself at that point, but it would have been slow moving. I moved around slowly and carefully. I just didn't feel that great. If I tried to get up quickly, I would see "stars". That persisted for quite a while, it just gradually got less and less dramatic and took more and more exertion for it to happen as time passed.

Jimmy Golden. MY GOLDEN MIND, A JOURNEY THROUGH EPILEPSY AND BRAIN SURGERY

Before I knew it, we were heading down to have my staples removed. It felt good. The area where the incision was itched a little, so when she removed the staples, it felt great. It didn't hurt at all whatsoever. She told me to continue to put ointment on it and it would keep the scar from becoming big or noticeable. It isn't either. I completely shave my whole head, and most people never notice it. I must point it out for most people to even see it. I was very surprised how subtle it ended up being. It doesn't bother me at all. The surgeon did a wonderful job.

I ended up, after living in my house for several years, finally officially meeting the man who lives across the street from me. His name is Bill. We ended up becoming friends. We had a common interest because he is a retired cop. I had always had the suspicion he was a police officer just by looking at him. I told him that after I met him and he told me he gets that all the time. I actually frequently get that too. So maybe it's true that people who work in those fields do have something about the way they look. Anyway, he told me that if I ever needed anything to make sure and let him know. We told him about my situation. My parents told him that it made them feel good that he lived across the street from us. I am glad he lives there too honestly. It makes me feel better knowing he is there when Christina is home alone.

A little over a month after my parents arrived, and I was feeling good enough, they decided it was time for them to head back to Oregon. We were sad, but we couldn't expect them to stay forever. We said our goodbyes and wished them a safe drive. We thanked them for everything. I gave my Dad a shirt before he left. It is a shirt that I had my friend get from my work that you can't get from anywhere else. It was the only way I could think of to try and thank him for all that they did. A sort of symbol. He did something for me that nobody else could have done, so I did something for him that nobody else could. He worked there for twenty-five years before retiring recently, so I think he appreciated it. They told us, if we needed them, they would come back in a second, and all we had to do is tell them. We gave them hugs and they headed home.

It was time for me to start being on my own during the day. It was weird. But I managed. I spent a lot of time with

Oliver, our Yorkie. I watched a lot of TV. I couldn't do too much. I was still not feeling all that great. I mean, I was feeling much better, I just couldn't do much that was physical. If I did anything that required physical exertion, it made me see stars and feel like I wanted to pass out. The doctors encouraged me to go on walks. Nobody really thought it was a good idea for me to be walking around on my own yet though. So, Aldo, like he always does, offered to help. He told me he would stop by after work several days a week to walk with me. We started doing that for a while, which was nice. I got to get some exercise, and hang out with Aldo at the same time. Around that same time, I also went with him and had my first post op sushi!

Bill, the retired cop from across the street, had noticed I had been going for walks with Aldo, and told me that if I ever needed a walking partner, to let him know. He said he was "always up for a good stroll". I ended up taking him up on his offer one day. Before I knew it, Bill and I became friends, and we started walking together regularly, several times a week. I am glad Bill lives across the street, he really helped me get through the time I spent off work. We spent a good amount of time hanging out, playing with Oliver, watching TV, going for walks, and going out to lunch. He would drive me to places I needed to go from time to time. Bill is a great man, and he ended up becoming a big part of my journey.

I started going to my post op visits with my surgeon not long after my surgery. As I said before, my appreciation for him only grew stronger after the operation. He really does treat his patients as a continuously growing family, and it didn't take me long to realize that. The visits with my surgeon were always similar in the beginning. The nurse would bring myself, and the person that drove me down to see him to the room. It was typically Ray at that point in the process. I would sit with my green notebook filled with all the questions that I had lined up for him, and we would patiently wait for him to come in. He would enter the room, always casually, with a big smile on his face. "Jimmy! How are you doing buddy!?" I would tell him I was doing good. He would come over and shake my hand, and then shake Ray's hand and ask how he was doing. He would pull up a chair, and then get straight to it. "So, any seizures?" I would tell him the good news. "Nope!" He would put on a big smile again, every time, and stick out his fist to give me a fist bump and say "Alright! That's what I like to hear!" Or something of that nature. He would then give Ray a fist bump too. He must be one of the most down to earth people I have ever met. He would always ask what kind of questions I had for him. I would ask away, and he would answer away. Everything was good though. I really didn't have anything of substance, I just asked him things out of curiosity. He did help me though. My surgeon helped keep me on track through all of this. He helped me keep my head up. He answered emails, he gave me advice if I asked him for it. He was never too busy for me. He really is a great man. He was nothing like my childhood brain surgeon stereotypes made me think he would be.

Before I knew it, it had been almost four months since surgery. It was coming up on May! I couldn't believe it! I had seen my surgeon a couple of times, and was due to see my epileptologist. After the surgery, I was placed off work for recovery until around the middle of April. It was apparent that wasn't going to work. I was still feeling like I was going to pass out when I did anything mildly strenuous, and was seeing stars if

Jimmy Golden. MY GOLDEN MIND, A JOURNEY THROUGH EPILEPSY AND BRAIN SURGERY

I got up too quickly, or moved too fast. I wasn't complaining though, because I was seizure free!!! What a feeling!!! No seizures!!! When I saw the epileptologist, I told her how I was feeling, and I asked her what she thought. I told her I had been walking a lot, trying to work through it, and had been using my exercise bike in my bedroom. She asked me "Do you have a particular date you are trying to be completely healed by?" I told her I didn't. I knew what she was getting at. She told me I didn't have anything to prove to anyone, including myself. She said that I had a serious operation on my brain, and I needed to let it heal on its own, and I needed to take it easy. She told me I was doing what lots of people tend to do in my situation, and was trying to push myself to get better, which is not right. I needed to allow myself to get better naturally, and accept the time it takes. I appreciated what she told me. I think I needed to hear it. I was pushing too hard, and I was being too hard on myself. She told me she was going to put me out of work until July 17, 2017. Walking was fine, but if I didn't feel good, I needed to rest. No heavy lifting, exercise or otherwise. Take it easy. Enjoy myself. I had what seems to be a successful surgery so far, be happy and relax. I really like her. She is an amazing person, and she is so sweet and insightful. She really knows exactly how to talk to people. I took her advice to heart.

So, still being off work, I had lots of time on my hands. More time with Oliver. That was always nice. It was honestly hard on me though. Being alone that much was difficult. I was thankful that my friends like Aldo, Ron, Bill, Chris and Maira, Scott, everyone in general, were around to get me out of the house. I don't think I would have made it through everything in one piece without them. Even being seizure free isn't a cure all. I still have a hard time sometimes honestly. I never know if another seizure is right around the corner. I never had a seizure trigger. I am one of the people I spoke of at the beginning of this book that always felt like prey, being silently stalked by a monster who lives inside you. A monster that is ready and willing to strike whenever it sees fit, silently torturing you with its unpredictability. If I may use another metaphor here, surgery may have "washed away" the dirt, grease and soil that were the seizures caused by my epilepsy, but, I am still stained. It never fully went away. It left its mark on me. With the beauty and wonder that is life, that stain may, and I believe will, slowly fade away over time, but, for now, it persists. The main problem is that the fear still shakes me to my core. Déjà vu told me a seizure had begun. So, when I see something familiar, I feel a slight sense of dread, and I wonder, if only for a minute, "is this it? Is this the day my neurosurgery fails? Is this my first post brain surgery seizure?" Eventually, all familiar things so far have become just that. Familiar things, and I move on, seizure free, carrying my stain, but living life, enjoying life, happy, still learning to cope, and wondering when that fear will pass. I am still only learning though. I do struggle a little to deal with that fear. It is gripping me less and less, and I am battling it. I have overcome great odds in the past. I have persevered. I will find a way to wash that stain away. I want to carry nothing but a scar and a fountain of knowledge. I intend to use my experience to help people who are looking for someone with answers, like I once was. I was once there. I know how it feels to look for someone who has experienced what I have gone through. Hoping to find someone who has experienced the things you are going to go through. Hoping they can answer questions nobody else can possibly answer. I know how it feels to be in the darkness, but I found a way out, once upon a time.

When my friends were busy, I stayed at home most of the time, by myself, with Oliver, my little pup, honestly, feeling sad from medications, hoping desperately that the monster that lives inside of me wouldn't strike again. Always hoping, but never knowing for sure, that the surgeon removed what once seemed to live within my haunted mind. In a way, it made me feel as though I was never really alone. I know that sounds kind of creepy, but it is true, and it still is.

My little sister Brittany came over with her son Jason one day to visit and spend some time with us. She hung out for a few days. That was very cool. It broke up some of the monotony of being at home alone, on disability, without a driver's license. Plus, obviously, I enjoy their company. We decided when she was visiting, we were going to surprise my Mom for Mother's Day, and fly the three of us up to Oregon. We worked it out with my Dad and older sister Jennifer, who also lives up there close to my parents. Her and my Dad would pretend they were going to a

Jimmy Golden. MY GOLDEN MIND, A JOURNEY THROUGH EPILEPSY AND BRAIN SURGERY

bee conference, because my sister was going to start keeping bees, and they would really go pick us up at the airport. My Mom would stay at my sister Jennifer's house for the day and babysit her kids, while her husband Joe was at work. It was a good plan. So, we put it into play.

Brittany came over the night before, and stayed the night at my house with her son Jason. In the morning, we headed off to see, who Jason calls "far away Grandma". It all worked out according to plan. We stayed up there for a week. We completely surprised my Mom. She had no idea. It was great. Brittany, Jason and I stayed at my parent's house. On Mother's Day itself, Jennifer and her family came over, and so did my grandparents. It was a nice day. I wrote my Mom a letter as a gift, and it is a true story of course. I framed it, and in the bottom of it, I placed a piece of shattered reflector behind the glass with the letter. You will understand why when you read what I wrote. I gave that to her as her Mother's Day gift. Here is what I wrote:

I went for a walk today, along a path I have taken many times before. I used to run it before epilepsy entered my life,

Jimmy Golden. MY GOLDEN MIND, A JOURNEY THROUGH EPILEPSY AND BRAIN SURGERY

while training for the academy that epilepsy stole. Christina and I have jogged side by side together, laughing, teasing and racing one another, all while racing the clock and trying to best our fastest time on that set course. Recently, of course, things haven't been quite the same. Instead of running and jogging for cardio fitness, the exercise has turned into walking for joint health and blood flow while recovering from brain surgery. There have been many changes these past couple of years. There is no doubt about that. Sometimes, it seems, very little is the same. Today, though, I was unexpectedly reminded of one thing that hasn't changed over the years. While walking, I looked down, and saw a familiar sight. I had a slight feeling of déjà vu, but not the kind that used to send me spiraling down the rabbit hole of a seizure. It was, after all I have been through with seizures these past couple of years, what I can imagine a normal person experiences when they say they have had déjà vu. I saw a shattered piece of reflector on the ground in the dirt. The thing is, I used to walk this route before surgery, alone. I remember putting on my medical alert bracelet in the mornings before my walks, hoping it was an unnecessary task, but never really knowing. One day,

Jimmy Golden. MY GOLDEN MIND, A JOURNEY THROUGH EPILEPSY AND BRAIN SURGERY

while out on my walking route, I had my most significant complex partial seizure while away from home and alone. With unlikely odds, the seizure began the typical storm of déjà vu in my mind at the same moment that I looked down at that very same shattered reflector. Déjà vu was something I had unfortunately become accustomed to by that point in my life with the vast amount of seizure activity my brain had experienced up to that point. I remember the familiarity of that reflector as if it had belonged to me my whole life. Next, a car passed me with an advertisement on its side and I "recognized it". Not the advertisement... the situation. Then another car passed with a person who I felt I "knew". Then, the pattern of the birds in the air became familiar. Next, the song on my iPod seemed to become connected to the time and place I was standing and the football equipment on the field and the next car coming down the road transitioned, in my mind, all to things already experienced in my past. I noticed the familiarity of the temperature of the air on my skin. Then, my eyes went back to the reflector. The feeling of déjà vu was becoming overwhelming at that point and seemed to be the only reality left to focus on, because at that point in the

Jimmy Golden. MY GOLDEN MIND, A JOURNEY THROUGH EPILEPSY AND BRAIN SURGERY

seizure, it is all absorbing. You are not lucky enough to have crossed the threshold into being cognitively unaware due to the seizure, but you seem to be trapped in the sort of mental darkness no man's land that is caused by it. You have lost most cognitive function and can only really comprehend and focus on the overwhelming sensations that have overridden your nervous system and have hijacked your conscious being. So, you ride it out, like the hundreds of times before. You fight to maintain control of not only your body functions but your mind, hoping, with the small piece of your cognitive awareness that perseveres through the electrical storm, that it won't become another one of "those". Another... dare you even think its name while it's happening in case it triggers it somehow? A tonic clonic. I had hoped the Sheriff I walked by parked in the school parking lot would notice, or that someone would see me lying in the dirt and flag him down if it went full blown. The déjà vu spells like that all seem like sort of a replay from another time of your life. Then, suddenly the sensational rush of the seizure sets in and what cognition I had been managing to hold on to, without me knowing, slipped away. Next thing I remember, I was up the

Jimmy Golden. MY GOLDEN MIND, A JOURNEY THROUGH EPILEPSY AND BRAIN SURGERY

road, confused and wandering aimlessly and caught myself gripping my left-hand open and closed over and over, my dead giveaway for a complex partial seizure. Fortunately, I was able to gather myself, I hadn't wandered into traffic, and my medical bracelet was never needed that day. Thankfully, so far, because of the help of my support system, my doctors and neurosurgery, I may never need it. Today though, when I saw that reflector, I wasn't reminded of epilepsy or seizures, I was reminded of my Mother. I didn't think of wandering confused next to the high school in a postictal state. I was reminded of my Mother feeding me pudding in ICU after brain surgery because she knew that's all I could keep down. I remembered her making me omelets at home after being discharged from the hospital, with salt of course, because I was too weak to make them myself, and of her making sure I got my medications on time, every time. I remembered her trying to be strong and hide her feelings the night before and the day of surgery, even though I knew she was scared. I remembered the daily texts from her to make sure I am doing well and don't need anything. I remember her telling me she will fly down to help me at a moment's notice if I need her. I remembered that, at 30 years old, going on 31, and going through the roughest patch of my life, my Mom is still my Mother, and that she is still there to take care of me when I need her, like she has always been, even when it isn't easy. I remembered that, not only has that not changed, but it never will. Thank you for everything Mom, not just for the help and support these past tough couple of years, but for these past 31 and on. Happy Mother's Day.

May 14, 2017

I had hoped that by writing her that letter, that maybe I could give her an idea of how thankful I was for everything she had done for me. My Mom is a wonderful person, and I don't just say that because she is my Mother. She is a caretaker at heart, and she really helped us in our time of need.

I slowly continued to get better after I got home from our trip to see my mother. It didn't happen overnight, but the progression was there. I continued to walk with Bill. I tried to keep myself busy. I tried to keep my mind occupied. I tried to stay positive so I wouldn't let the medications get to me. The

Jimmy Golden. MY GOLDEN MIND, A JOURNEY THROUGH EPILEPSY AND BRAIN SURGERY

Epileptologist told me if I stay seizure free for two years after surgery, my brain activity will be tested with an EEG. If it is normal, she will start to taper me off the medications slowly. They do not want to risk causing a seizure by starting to taper medications too early, which is understandable to me. Honestly, the medications are becoming more tolerable. I think that over time, my body is becoming more and more used to them. The side effects, like the down moods and slow thinking, are becoming less and less noticeable as time passes, to the point where it rarely bothers me. I am hoping to get off them one day though, obviously.

When my potential return to work date came around, as much as I was dying to go back to work, I wasn't ready. I was sad, because I really wanted to go back. I was sick and tired of being at home. I wanted to work, but I was still feeling light headed and seeing stars when I did things that were at all strenuous. The doctors told me that it was normal for that to happen, and wanted me to take it easy a little longer. They said it was just a blood flow issue. It was nothing to be concerned about, it just takes time. My job involves physical labor, and heights, so I didn't blame them. I knew I wasn't ready. The doctor pushed my date back until august 21st. I ended up having an appointment scheduled with my primary neurologist to talk it over with him and see where we stood at that point. In the meantime, though, I had reached my six-month mark of seizure freedom! July 17th, 2017. On that day, in the state of California, I became eligible to request to have my driving privileges reinstated! What a big day!

I brought the necessary paperwork for my driver's license to the medical insurance/paperwork office of my neurologist. He had told me because I had been seizure free for so long, he no longer felt I was a risk behind the wheel! He told me he would be happy to fill out the paperwork. He filled it out, and soon after I got a call to pick it up. Bill drove me to the office to pick it up, and I faxed it to the driver's safety branch of the DMV at the location where my case was located within the DMV system. I talked to them on the phone to make sure everything was squared away. By talking to them, I was pretty sure, if they gave it back, it was going to be a several month's long process. At least it was in the works now! It had been almost two years since I had driven a vehicle. Driving has always meant a lot to me. I am a car guy. Losing my license was devastating to me. They told me, basically, I would hear back from them in the mail within about four to six weeks, telling me if they needed more paperwork or not, and what the next step would be. Then I would receive a phone call, telling me if they wanted to do an over the phone or a in person interview. I would have to do that. Then they would convene their panel, review my paperwork from the neurologist and all my medical history. From there, they would make their decision based on everything, and then decide if they wanted me to take another behind the wheel, if they thought I was safe to drive again. Oh yeah, I decided this was going to be Months! I mailed the letter late July 2017.

My neurology appointment came around. The extra time they gave me off did me wonders! I was feeling much better! I had decided, unless the doctor told me otherwise, I was ready to get my old life back, I was ready to go back to work! It had been almost seven months since surgery now, and I was feeling good to go! No more stars, no more feeling like I was going to pass out or feeling light headed while doing anything strenuous. I thought that going back to work would really improve my mood. I really wanted this. I really had a feeling it would put some light back in me. I really felt it was time. I was still seizure free. My life had been completely turned around by the surgery. No more seizures, no more depersonalization, no nothing. I felt wonderful.

Christina and I went into the room with the neurologist. He asked me how I was feeling. I told him I was feeling better. He told me he was happy to see me, and it was good to hear that. As always, he asked if I had any seizures, I told him no, and he told me that was great news. He asked me if I thought I needed any more time to recover, or how was I feeling. I told him I thought I was ready! I was good to go. I wanted to go back to work! He was happy for me, and was happy to send me back to work. I would return full duty on August 21st, 2017. It was set. It was incredible. My recovery was over.

Chapter 13. Moving on.

I had been off work for one year, ten months and seventeen days total before I returned to work. It was a long road, but it was going to be good to walk back in. I missed my job. I was a little nervous, because I wake up at 3:30 am for work. I had become used to getting up at around 9:00am. It was going to take some time to get used to the swing of things again. I had also been off so long, recovering from a surgery, and not doing anything very physical, that when I started doing physical labor, I knew it would be hard on me.

Jimmy Golden. MY GOLDEN MIND, A JOURNEY THROUGH EPILEPSY AND BRAIN SURGERY

The waking up was nowhere near as bad as I thought it would be. For some reason, I got right back used to it. Well, about as acclimated to as you ever get to getting up at 3:30 am anyway. I was sore. It felt good to start doing some work though. I could tell that it was good for my mind. I was instantly happier. It felt great to see people I hadn't seen in so long. I missed people. Not only some of the people I like, but just being around people in general. It really did feel good to be back. Work is good for you, I believe, both mentally and physically. I know it does wonders for my mind. I felt much happier being back at work.

I work a four tens shift. Monday through Thursday. Aldo had been driving me to work. He told me he had no problem driving me for as long as it takes. He works for the same company, and he lives in the next neighborhood over. It's not out of his way, but I really appreciated it. He is so good to me. I really would have had a lot more difficult of a time through all of this without Aldo. Not just him, but he played a huge role in the success of my story. I could rattle off a thank you list like an academy award speech... Ron, Ray, my parents, Bill, the doctors

Jimmy Golden. MY GOLDEN MIND, A JOURNEY THROUGH EPILEPSY AND BRAIN SURGERY

(obviously), Christina, Chris, Maira, Scott, Darren, my sisters, Nick…. Even the president helped me out mentally by sending me that letter. The people in my life are what got me through all of this in one piece. That is my point. Don't forget that. Focus on the people around you. Don't allow yourself to get secluded. Don't shut yourself out or don't allow the person with epilepsy in your life to shut himself or herself out if it's not you. People are the key to success. You, or they won't make it alone. Also, the people that are connected to someone with epilepsy are greatly impacted by the person with epilepsy. It can be very difficult on them also, they can't be overlooked either, although it's important to remember it isn't the person with epilepsy's fault. If you don't have it, and you know someone who does, always remember that. They didn't ask for epilepsy. Never allow yourself to begin to resent them. Resentment is a crushing feeling. This is about everyone. People helping people is what makes things work, it's what makes things happen, its why my story is such a success.

    I got home at the end of my first week back at work. It was a great week. I went through a bunch of training mostly.

Nothing major. When I got home, I relaxed for a bit. I decided I better check the mail. While on my way back from the mail box, I looked through the envelopes and I got to one that caught my attention. It was for me, and it was from the DMV driver's safety division. I got inside and I went in and sat on the bed. I didn't notice until this very second while writing this, but I sat in the very same spot where I opened the Obama letter. I opened it to see what the next step was going to be. I was really worried they were going to want a bunch of paperwork. Again, just like with the letter from the President, I was blown away. It informed me that the actions taken on the day that my license was suspended had been overturned, and that I was able to go to the nearest DMV office to have my driver's license renewed. That was it. It was done. They approved it already. I was getting my driver's license back. The same week I got to go back to work. Seven months seizure free. I honestly felt emotional. I couldn't remember the last time I felt so happy. What a privilege. Those doctors really had changed my life completely. I told Christina. We both put our hands in the air in celebration and she ran over and gave me a hug and a kiss. She called her dad and told him the news. She asked him if he could drive me to the DMV the next day to get it, because he was off, and of course, he did.

After I renewed my license, Ray dropped me off at home. Christina was still at work. My truck had insurance on it through Christina's plan, but I was listed as a non-driver because I had the suspension, so I couldn't drive my truck at all even though I was now newly licensed again. I needed to get it insured properly first. I called around, but people wanted outrageous amounts of money because of the medical suspension, which I thought seemed insane, and possibly illegal because of the Americans with disabilities act, but I am not sure yet. I may have to research that. The insurance company I had insurance with prior to the suspension was going to just about triple my insurance rate to nearly 3,000.00 a year for just my 2007 model truck alone, with a perfectly clean driving record. The insurance companies do not consider the difference between different types of suspensions, and therefore charge someone with a disability a higher rate for insurance than someone without because their license had been medically suspended at no fault of their own, even if their driving record is perfectly clean. The Americans with disabilities act states that an insurance company may not charge a person with a disability more than someone else, solely because they have a disability. The insurance companies look for loopholes to exploit though, and it seems they possibly use the medical suspensions as one of those loopholes, or so it seems to me anyway, but I am no lawyer. Frustrating. I was deemed safe to drive not only by my neurologist but also the driver's safety board of the DMV. The suspension was medical and precautionary only. So, why was I being treated the same as someone who had a suspension for reckless driving incidents, DUI issues, or other disciplinary reasons? I was no longer being considered a risk to anyone. I was not happy. The insurance companies were labeling my medical suspension as a "conviction", although my driving record shows no convictions.

All frustrations aside, I needed to get insurance, and I wanted it that day. After calling around, and feeling like the rates being offered were all unfair and bias against me with my previous medical suspension, I decided I wanted to go talk to an insurance company in town, in person, so I talked to Bill to see if he wanted to go with me. He was relaxing that day, so he offered to let me drive his car instead of him going. I really appreciated that and took him up on it. So, after almost two years of not driving, my first-time driving was driving Bill's car. After pulling out of the driveway, I turned on his radio, and the song "Sweet Emotion" was playing on the radio. Very fitting for the situation.

It was an amazing feeling, being behind the wheel of a car again. Sure, I wasn't flying down a drag strip in a full caged race car like I used to. Nonetheless, it was just as satisfying as it used to be for me when I would blow through the finish line in my old 1965 big block nova race car, engine howling, passing through the beams at 125 mph. I ended up buying insurance that day when I drove Bills car, and had to pay extra for my suspension. Everyone was charging for it. I shopped around, but I couldn't find a reputable insurance company that didn't charge.

I have found that living with epilepsy can be sort of that way. At least it feels that way sometimes. I have had to make a conscious effort to not get in that kind of mind set. Fight the temptation to feel like "everything that could possibly go wrong, always does". When all of this first started, it was very easy to fall into the "why me" trap. You must be careful with that. It isn't easy to get out of. The thing is, if you really think about it, you can make that argument about anything. As humans in general though, most of the time, we only seem to make it when something has gone terribly wrong for us. Some deep thinkers may, but in general, people don't seem to. It doesn't really make sense to make it otherwise. I mean, if I won some money on a scratcher, I wouldn't be asking myself, "why me?" So, why ask when I get an unlikely disorder? Is it simply because we don't want the negative situation? That seems to be the logical answer. The point is, it is an unanswerable question, at least in many of the cases of epilepsy. So, focusing on it can only do you or your loved one's harm. Everyone is better off learning to accept epilepsy for what it is. Make informed decisions about what you want to do about it. Are you going to pursue treatment? Are you going to become active and vocal about it? Are you afraid? When I learned I had epilepsy, I wanted out of the game. I didn't want to have seizures forever. If there was any way at all not to have them, I was interested. I doubt many people do want them. I would say nobody does, but you never know. I worked in a prison, and I have met some strange characters in my day. I wouldn't be surprised if someone out there exists who wants to have seizures somewhere. Anyway, I did research about the topic, like I always do about everything, and I knew surgery could be possibly be an option. I didn't know for sure if it would be an option for me, but when my epileptologist asked me, after all the "episodes" I had been suffering through for so long at that point, I knew the answer right away. I didn't have hesitation.

I felt as though I could see a "light at the end of the tunnel" after my epileptologist asked me about surgery. I finally had some real hope that my seizures could one-day end. I did a lot of reading on online forums from people who had been through this kind surgery before. I read both good and bad things that people had written about their surgeries, the process involved to get to that point, and the aftermath. I tried to find books to read on the subject written in the first-person perspective from someone who had lived it but did not have any success. That is part of the reason I am here. As far as the "finding both good and bad experiences go", I encourage you to not be deterred by people's negative comments who post things online. It can be easy to get caught up in things like that, but the reality is, anyone can post anything online, and some people, especially when caught in a dark place, like the one epilepsy may put them in, may not end up offering the best advice. Some people have a natural distaste for anything medical related, and no matter what experience they may have had, will perceive it as having been negative. Subconscious bias can be a powerful thing, and can make things seem much worse than they really are, or were, for some people. I can tell you from my own personal experience, from start to finish through my journey with epilepsy, it has been an up and down, sometimes dark, frequently rough, sometimes sad, but sometimes happy road. The highlights and bright shining stars along it have been the people that have helped me navigate it. The medical treatment I was open to receiving is what enabled me to make it to an end. I chose to ignore the negativity I read, and take a chance. I reached my hand out of the dark world in which I was stuck, back into the light. I hoped to find people who would be able to pull me out, and people were there to do just that. I was pulled from the darkness of epilepsy on January 19, 2017. My support system helped keep me stable along the way, and the advanced science and the trained professionals working in the field of neurology and neurosurgery changed my life by ending my seizures, and for that, I will be forever grateful.

Jimmy Golden. MY GOLDEN MIND, A JOURNEY THROUGH EPILEPSY AND BRAIN SURGERY

Chapter 14. Final thoughts.

As I said in the beginning, everyone's experience with epilepsy is somewhat different. Nobody's is precisely the same. We all have similarities though, and we all have one thing in common, we have seizures. Well, thanks to some incredible people, I no longer do, as of January 19, 2017. Well that's not true, my last seizure was two days before surgery. January 17th. As I said before, I kept a log of all my seizures from a certain point on. I started that log on October 11th of 2015. By that point, I was already fully medicated on the medication the hospital had given me, which slowed my seizure activity way down to about one a week or so on average, but sometimes more. From October

Jimmy Golden. MY GOLDEN MIND, A JOURNEY THROUGH EPILEPSY AND BRAIN SURGERY

11th, 2015, to January 17th, 2017, I logged eighty-eight seizures in my log book, and those were the ones I knew of. Sometimes I had seizures and didn't realize it. I had to be told, so it is possible I missed some. I really started having seizures about a year before that, and was having up to ten a day before medication. I have always figured my best guess is that I have had somewhere in the ball park of around eight hundred or so seizures. That may sound like a lot to some people, and it may sound like nothing to others. That is my journey though. I thought it may be interesting, and fitting to add my last seizure entry from my log book, into this book. So here it is.

Monday January 17 at approx. 5:00 pm

While reading a news article about president Obama and his family completing an escape room, I had a typical type of seizure for me, seemed to be a complex partial. I started feeling some signs of déjà vu. I tried to ignore it and keep reading, but it got worse and progressed into the full seizure feelings I get. I then waited what seemed like a couple minutes until it was over and I left the room where I was reading, and

Jimmy Golden. MY GOLDEN MIND, A JOURNEY THROUGH EPILEPSY AND BRAIN SURGERY

went and laid down and relaxed on the couch because I felt very tired. When Christina got home, she knew I had a seizure by the look on my face she said, as usual. I didn't feel well for a while afterwards.

Please excuse the lack of depth and clarity in the log. I wrote it in a post-ictal state. I wanted to put it in the book exactly as it is in my log. I thought it was kind of cool that, after getting my letter from the president, my very last seizure happened while reading an article about him and his family. Funny coincidence. Some of my logs are more in depth than that, but they are all simple. I only got somewhat more in depth if the seizure had a lot of depth to it, or if there was something I felt needed to be noted about it. Something out of the ordinary, things like that.

I know what you or your family or friend is going through, at least to a certain extent. It is hard. It sucks, put plainly. It's hard on the person with epilepsy first and foremost, its hard on everyone involved with that person. It's just hard in general. No matter who you are in the situation though, you can make it through. Fight the fight. Go to battle against epilepsy. Don't succumb to it. Find the people who matter. People are the key to success. Family, friends, doctors, surgeons, coworkers, people at sandwich shops who remember what you like on your sandwich. It is people who are going to help with you or your loved one's epilepsy. Really listen to what people say to you, and the ones who don't have good things to say, separate from them. The ones who help, keep them close and appreciate them dearly.

It's funny really, epilepsy kind of did something for me. In a way, it added a new flavor to life. I know that it is a bit of a cliché, but going through everything I have been through, all the darkness, the trauma. It really made me see what is important in life, at least for me. I really care less about "stuff" in general. I don't "want" as much as I used to. I don't "need" to go out and buy the new cool thing, or this or that. My paid off 2007 model truck is more than sufficient for me. I see the beauty in things more than I used to. I have always been artistic and have valued things of that nature, but I do so now more than ever. Now though, I notice squirrels in the trees playing, or children in the park with smiles on their faces, and things like that make me happy, when before, they were just animals and random kids. I notice the lyrics more in music, and how they relate to my life, and I feel the emotion in the music on a deeper level, when before, music was just something I rocked out to while passing time in my truck. I mean don't get me wrong, I always loved music, it's just deeper now. Life just seems a little more meaningful since I started battling epilepsy. I can almost appreciate epilepsy in a way because of that. I used to be a bit of a pessimist, I can admit that. My glass was typically half empty. I don't feel that way anymore. I don't know if other people have noticed this change or not, but I hope so. If not, try. Try and find it. Try and notice the world around you. Not everything is wrong. We may be different in a way, but that is okay, we can persevere. Humans are terrific at adaptation.

I remember when I decided to write this book. I was at a post op visit with my surgeon. Ray had taken me down. We left very early, so we got there almost an hour early, but we decided we might as well go in. I checked in and we sat in the waiting room. Always better early than late. I have a tremendous amount of respect for my surgeon, especially by that point, I was seizure free after all, he treated me like a family member. There was no way I was going to make him wait. We were only there a couple minutes and he came out into the waiting room and waived at us. "What's up Jimmy!?" We waved back and said hello from across the room. That was a particularly good visit. We took pictures together that day. I had my picture with my surgeon custom framed by the company that sponsors my artwork, and I have it proudly hanging in my office. I am looking at it right now. We both have big smiles on our faces, and our arms around each other's shoulders, like old, longtime friends, not a surgeon and patient. That is who my surgeon is. He is incredible.

A couple minutes later he came back out. He walked up to us and asked me if I would mind if he introduced me to a few people. I told him of course not. He had changed my life after all, I would do anything for that man I could. He introduced me to two parents of kid. He told them that I had the same surgery that their kid may be having, if they decided to proceed. He showed them my scar, and explained a few things to them. He told them what he could without giving them any of my medical information. I looked at him and said, "You tell them anything you want about my medical record." He said "really? Are you sure?" I said "absolutely".

He talked to them a little and told them a little about the minor differences between a few things, and he asked if they would like to speak with me, and if that would be okay with me. I told them I would be happy to talk to them about anything they would like to know. They said they would love to talk to me. He told us he had to run to go see another patient and left us to talk.

They began talking to me and asking about the process and how it felt, what it was like, if I was seizure free, how the surgery was, how I felt about the surgeon. Lots of things. I was happy to give them all of the information they asked for. They were scared parents, worried about putting their child under the knife, but also worried about not making the decision, and letting him continue to have seizures when he possibly had the opportunity to finally become seizure free. I told them the same thing I will tell you as the reader.

Jimmy Golden. MY GOLDEN MIND, A JOURNEY THROUGH EPILEPSY AND BRAIN SURGERY

Before I had my temporal lobectomy, I had always said having Lasik was the best thing I had ever done for myself. Now, having brain surgery, by far, blows that out of the water. I would, without a doubt, do it again in a second if I needed to. It was the single greatest decision I have ever made. It changed the entire course of my life. I am thankful every day that I responded "yes" that day when my epileptologist called. It honestly is nothing to be afraid of. The risks are minimal, and the pain is very tolerable. It really doesn't last that long. Sure there is some, but it is more than tolerable. Sure, you don't feel good in the hospital, but you get the flu during your life too, you can't avoid that either. At least with this, you have great odds of changing your life forever! If you or your loved one is thinking about getting an operation like this done, I would recommend going for it. The science behind it is great. It is impressive. Don't be afraid. Fight the battle. Take it on.

After talking with them, they thanked me. They told me I had made them feel much better about the situation. They had been very uneasy up until that point. I imagine it must be hard on parents, especially not being able to talk to someone who had been through it themselves. Not being able to see living proof that it works. I knew first hand that it is either extremely hard or impossible to find books written in the first person from someone who has epilepsy and has gone through brain surgery. It made me feel good to help those people. I wasn't going back to corrections, I wouldn't likely be able to be a street cop, and I wanted to find a way to help people. I realized right then and there, that day, although I didn't tell anyone, I was going to try and write this book. A book to show people what this process is like and that it is not what people might imagine. That it is worth it. Hopefully give some people the confidence they need to give it a shot. I wrote it to give advice. To tell people the things that would have helped me during my process. To try and provide the insight, and hopefully the comfort that I was looking for back then. Me, with only a high school diploma, and missing part of my brain. I was going to prove that people who have battled epilepsy, and people who have had part of their brain removed could still do things. They could still accomplish whatever they wanted. They could still write books. People with epilepsy can hold good jobs. They can write letters to the president and receive a response. They can get their driver's license back. They can make the decision, go through with brain surgery, and come out seizure free. Their possibilities are endless. The glass doesn't always have to be half empty because you or your loved one has epilepsy. It is a matter of perspective and how you handle things. It depends on how you get things done. I fought to keep the darkness at bay. You need to do the same. If you stop, you lose the battle. No matter if you are the person with epilepsy, or a loved one. No matter what you do when it comes to epilepsy, you don't want to give in, because if you do, you lose. Keep fighting. Find a way to make it through every day, and every night. I know they can grow long and cold. I know it can be a steep, difficult, uphill battle with epilepsy. Just remember, keep your light glowing, never let the darkness extinguish it completely. You need it to survive. Stay strong, stay positive, and go for it. Make it happen. The answers are out there. Seek them out like I did. Don't be afraid. People are awesome, and science is a beautiful thing. Now, if you will excuse me, my fiancée is waiting. We are off to get married, and I'm driving.

Jimmy Golden. MY GOLDEN MIND, A JOURNEY THROUGH EPILEPSY AND BRAIN SURGERY

Jimmy Golden. MY GOLDEN MIND, A JOURNEY THROUGH EPILEPSY AND BRAIN SURGERY

Jimmy Golden. MY GOLDEN MIND, A JOURNEY THROUGH EPILEPSY AND BRAIN SURGERY

Jimmy Golden. MY GOLDEN MIND, A JOURNEY THROUGH EPILEPSY AND BRAIN SURGERY

Made in the USA
San Bernardino, CA
18 April 2018